DREAMVERSE

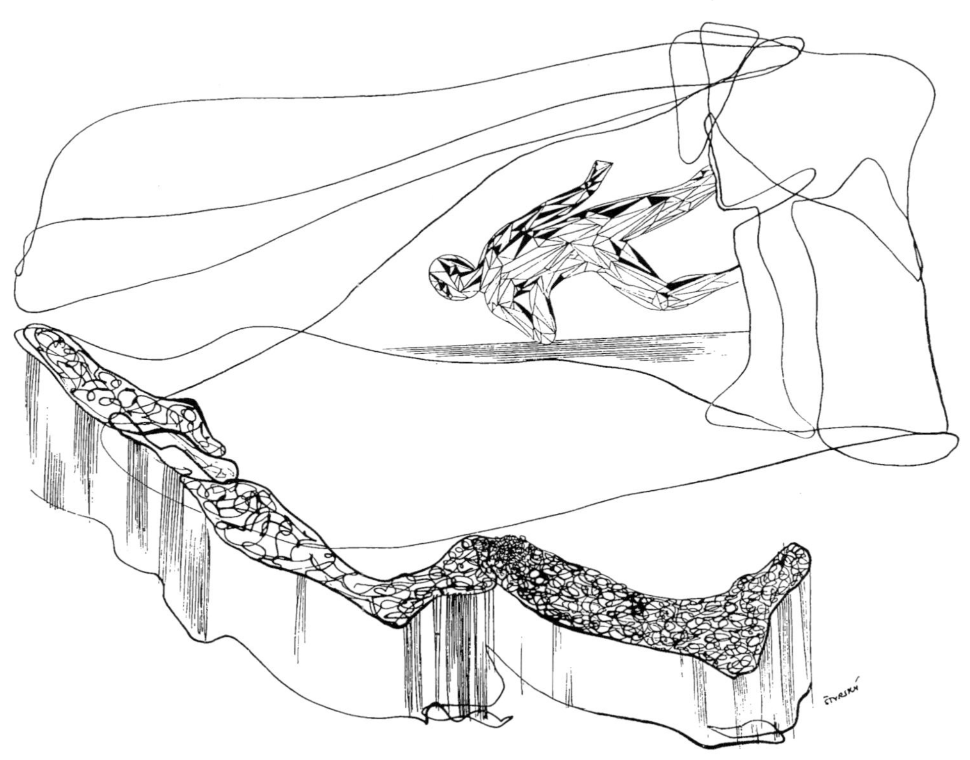

Flying Man, 1933, pen and ink on paper

Jindřich Štyrský

DREAMVERSE

Translated from the Czech by Jed Slast

TWISTED SPOON PRESS
PRAGUE
2018

ISBN 978-80-86264-38-7

The translation and publication of this book was made possible by a grant from the Ministry of Culture of the Czech Republic.

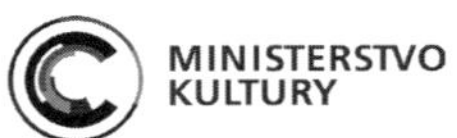

CONTENTS

VERSE

WRITINGS

INTRODUCTION

It would be futile to look for any concessions to what's in vogue or to outside pressures in Štyrský's work. The occupation and war have not diverted him from his path, which is at one with the path of revolution. Any dispassionate quest always serves the cause of humanity's complete liberation.

BENJAMIN PÉRET

Any points of contention in the discourse on the social function of art and its relation to reality and to the public cannot hope to be cleared up without a precise conceptual understanding of the nature of art's mission in all its historical mutability. To be sure, this activity of the spirit that we call art has witnessed over the past half century a shift no less seminal and revolutionary than the total transformation in how research is conducted in many scientific disciplines. Picasso and Apollinaire transformed the poetic universe so radically it was on a par with how Einstein transformed our view of the physical world and Freud our view of the psychic world. Modern art differs from the old masters in the same way astronomy differs from astrology. Poetry's revitalization is an evolutionary metamorphosis that has given rise to a new art, even if initiated in an era of a social system's degeneration. The work of art, having broken free of the servitude imposed on it by Church and State, took as its mission and purpose the emancipation of the human spirit. Poetry, therefore — and all spheres of art today are part and parcel of poetry — is a revolutionary force, if it is indeed authentic poetry : its liberating energy is inherent in its nature, in its inner wellsprings and specific methods, and when a poem employs heterogenous devices and betrays its own purpose, it reverts into its antithesis. Those who would reduce the complex dialectical relationship between art and reality to a relationship between the work of art and an external model requiring faithful representation would do well to remember what Baudelaire put to the doctrinaire's of realism : namely, if they know the whole of nature and all that reality holds, then they would know the inner life of man, for what happens in the inner world of a poet is no less real and no less important than all that occurs on the outside. Reality as depicted in paintings that copy nature is of life enfeebled and emasculated. In the high intensity of electro-poetic charges between the poles of subject and object, in the works of artists such as Goya, in which he became, in his own words, "completely distant from nature so that he could express in forms what he had experienced only in his imagination" and which surely are more revolutionary than the portraits of persons from aristocratic and plebeian classes, or Courbet, whose *The Dream* reveals the menacing power of one's inner nature, while in his landscapes nature is dead on arrival, the whole of reality incandesces and brims with feral life. Titian's *Sacred and Profane Love,* Giorgione's *The Tempest,* Bellini's *Four Allegories,* and Botticelli's *Primavera* have remained conundrums for art historians. Their message defies any conventional interpretation since it is poetry, that is, the transmutation of reality in the burning pyre of fantasy and dream. Poetry's relation to the world is not that of a mirror to the thing mirrored, but of an electric spark to combustible material. If the material is flammable enough and the spark strong enough, the combination of perception and imagination in the poem and the melding of poet and reader and viewer will produce an explosion. Poetry is an incandescent mode of life.

Jindřich Štyrský (born in Čermná, August 11, 1899—died in Prague, March 21, 1942) impacted the process of transforming painting from a representational mode into one identified with poetry through a method that was above all active and assertive. After debuting his early work in exhibitions held by the Student Society at the Academy of Fine Arts in Prague (1921–22), a larger group of early paintings displaying the morphology of late Cubism was exhibited in the first Devětsil Bazaar of Modern Art (1923 in Prague) : *Circus Simonette, The Singer, Black Pierrot* etc. Cubism for Štyrský during this period could be seen as a springboard to a new adventure. In the heady atmosphere of the avant-garde grouped together in Devětsil, Poetism became a fertile prelude to Surrealism. As F.X. Šalda has noted, Poetism initiated the faith in poetry's omnipotence, an act of faith in a single art with a thousand forms, a premonition of the universality of poetry, which is expressed one and the same both with means borrowed from other art forms — painting, sculpture, literature, theater, and music — and, especially, with new techniques, untainted by academic aesthetics and unlimited in their capacity to appropriate and invent. Štyrský included as well several photomontages and collages in the Bazaar exhibition, and they were the genesis of a new way to conceive the image, an intersection of verbal poetry and color poetry — the picture poem.

In 1925, Štyrský and Toyen left for Paris for three or four years. He had met Toyen in 1922, finding in her a companion to join him on his creative journey. While in Paris the poetry of color ripened in the work of both artists, which until Štyrský's death would resonate as a duet, each permeating the other without entirely merging, a two-in-one that made it virtually impossible to consider one apart from the other, a singular collaboration born of a deep friendship only death could cut short.

In the period that can be roughly dated to his leaving for Paris, Štyrský definitively turned away from Cubism. He now categorically renounced any sort of exterior a priori subject, the literal or free copying of which had been considered for centuries the painter's primary task. He arrived at a painting that was able to blossom in colors and lines on its own, independent of nature, that is, painting that has been labeled, albeit imprecisely, nonfigurative, abstract, or nonobjective art. The waning echoes of Cubism and its rigid geometry of planes vanished from Štyrský's work after *Landscape with Chessboard,* and the traditional techniques of the painter's craft were replaced by color sprayed across several objects and patterns situated on the canvas — tree leaves, matches, sugar cubes, the spiral of an apple peel — similar in method to that of the photogram (*Drowned Woman, Hoarfrost,* the series of lithographs for Vítězslav Nezval's poem *The Jewish Cemetery,* the drawings to *Maldoror,* etc.). The leaflet to Štyrsky and Toyen's Paris exhibition of their "ultraviolet paintings"* — which were as

* Cf. Karel Teige, "Ultrafialové obrazy čili artificielismus (Poznámky k obrazům Štyrského & Toyen)," *ReD*, vol. 1, no. 9 (1928), 315-317; English translation by Alexandra Büchler as "Ultraviolet Paintings, or, Artificialism (Notes on the Paintings of Štyrský & Toyen)," in *Between Worlds: A Sourcebook of Central European Avant-Gardes, 1910–1930* (Cambridge: MIT Press, 2002), 601–603. Teige states : "The Artificialist painting is a poem in the original Ancient Greek sense of the word for poetry, *poiesis,* that is, a supreme and independent creation. It is an independent, specific poem of color and line, not a reflection of a poem created by others and by different means. [...] Toyen and Štyrský make poetry by means of color and line in the same way Rimbaud's or Nezval's poetry is made with words."

if woven from quarter-tone streaks of mist, from vapors of nuance, from iridescent gossamer — proclaimed Artificialism, the pictorial twin of Poetism. Rather than a new ism, it was an impulse toward self-determination in the work of both artists at that moment in time, signaling their break with Cubism, which, according to the leaflet, still "viewed painting through the prism of a model, skewing reality instead of activating the imagination." It was thus a rejection of painting derived from an external model, a rejection of those "zaftig muses of a return to nature." Artificialism heralded the shift from an exterior to an interior model, and by precluding the forms of phenomenal reality, the painting became a representation of one's inner images.

Štyrský's gradual shift to Surrealism began in the early 1930s. There is no sharp dividing line between Artificialist and Surrealist painting. If Artificialism could be categorized as nonfigurative, so-called abstract art, then it presaged Surrealism in Štyrský's and Toyen's work, which began to display a perceptible evolution from the abstract to the concrete. From color and line that had lost attachment to phenomenal reality and did not interpret an external subject, objects slowly began to take on form, objects born in the imagination and not existing in everyday reality, that is, fantastical objects with contours becoming ever more distinct and a plasticity ever more concrete. With Štyrský, the first hints of this shift toward reifying images from dream and fantasy are noticeable in *The Death of Orpheus* and *Acacias* (1931), in *Milan Nights* and in several untitled paintings (1931–32), in the large-scale canvas *From My Diary* (1933), and in a number of drawings between the years 1931 to 1934, until it ultimately becomes the predominant mode in the painting *Čerchov* (1934), the point at which his work fully entered the province of Surrealism. Although nonfigurative aspects persisted in more than one of his contemporaneous and slightly later paintings included in the first exhibition of the Surrealist Group of Czechoslovakia at Mánes Gallery in Prague (1934), also evident was the growing prevalence of concretized irrational motifs in an effort to make the painting an accurate record of the world of imagination and lend the forms contrived by fantasy the same plastic quality as the things around us. The erotic vision that couples two phantoms in *Man and Woman,* which have the materiality of models from natural history but bring to mind objective reality, an uncanny mollusk, an undersea figure, or anatomical specimen only insofar as required for them to assume a sexual symbolism, is projected in the *Roots* series onto forms seen in reality that are then interpreted in accord with this vision's desire. The objectifying and concretizing of fantastic visions, the representation of which adopts the authenticity of the tangible so that the painting becomes a realistic representation of an irreal object, a depiction of a fantastic object, further evolved to the point where the painting was no longer merely a realistic depiction of fantasy but a fantastical configuration of real objects, in other words, a fantastical reality subjected to the dictates of desire. This shift from the reified to the real, from the actualization of imagination to an imaginative reality, from the clustering of fantastical objects to the fantastical clustering of everyday objects, selected and juxtaposed by desire as a form of contrast, for example, to express and symbolize desire's hidden tension, was accelerated by a series of photographs and hyperbolic collages that should be considered more than experimental marginalia as they were critical for Štyrský's development. They are artworks in their own right, on an equal footing with his large-scale canvases. As so often in the annals of modern art, a distinct evolutionary impulse is apparent here, and it does not start with work created by traditional techniques (i.e., oil painting) but with freer, less encumbered techniques that eschew the legerdemain of brushstroke (illustrations, prints, collages, photography, decalcomania, etc.), which academic prejudice has either judged to be "artes minores" or categorically rejected as art at all. Štyrský's photographs have demonstrated the viability of the process whereby what's visualized in the imagination assumes the authenticity of the real as well as the converse : the transformation of stark reality rendered hyperrealistically into phantasms and phantoms.

Štyrský's paintings from his joint exhibition with Toyen in early 1938, the last time the public had an opportunity to see his work before his death, and several smaller pieces he still had time to create belong among the full-fledged triumphs of Surrealism. They are eloquent testimonials to the materialization of the fantastic, which is the linchpin of current developments. *The Omnipresent Eye, In Memoriam F. G. Lorca, The Trauma of Birth, Mundane Awakening, Melancholy, The Somnambulist's Muse, The Gift, Glade in Red Light, Homage to Marx, Mayakovsky's Vest, At the Grave,*

Maldoror, the series *Dreams,* and others — that whole bountiful harvest between 1936 and 1941 together with the photographs (in Jindřich Heisler's *On the Needles of these Days*) and the many collages confirm the words of André Breton that "surreality would be embodied in reality itself and would be neither superior nor exterior to it." The overwhelming reality of the fantastical and the phantom-like quality of reality puts pay to the claim that Surrealism is nothing but an escape into the mists of supernatural metaphysics. The paintings created by the imagination, first as arrangements of fantastical objects composed of real elements and now as compositions of fantastical configurations, oneiric still lifes, and bizarre tableaux of real objects systematically plotted against a background, show that Surrealist noetics recognize the existence and primacy of objective reality.

To understand the terms Surrealism and surreality, their context needs to be determined first, and it should not be taken as the absolute antithesis of realism and reality. In the panorama of contemporary art, Surrealism has many commonalities and overlaps with abstract art, something evident in Štyrský's work, too, while it is clearly the opposite of neorealist tendencies. And yet the Surrealist painting is not nonobjective and nonrepresentational. Whether a spontaneous painting or drawing where the contours of things fade into arabesques (automatism of creation), or a compulsive hallucinatory incarnation of imagination and dream (automatism of vision), it is always a rendering of an inner model, an expression of an interior reality merging with the objective world from which it has sprung and in turn transfigures. This facet of Surrealism is often called magic realism.

Sapped by a chronic heart disease, Jindřich Štyrský died in an apocalyptic age of murdered poets. The brute oppression with which obscurantism proscribed the poetic mindset animating his work as degenerate could only steel the courageous resolve of the avant-garde and solidify the union between the will for a liberated poetry and the will for a fully liberated human. Looking at Štyrský's whole body of work, from the first fumbling efforts to the bright *Paradise Lost,* which is appallingly close chronologically to his final, unfinished painting, the tragic mask of Maldoror, one might wonder what direction his work would have taken if it had not been so abruptly brought to a close. Unappreciated today, his work awaits the judgment of the future, and the sole objectively valid criterion for such a judgment derives from a historically evolved outlook, from determining the evolutionary stage of an artistic phenomenon and the ambit of its anticipation and participation in the development of artistic culture. An evaluation of a work's magnitude and significance must be undertaken to arrive at any conclusions about evolutionary process and sedulity, to determine if the work is endowed with a proactive, fecundating power and acts progressively to move the evolutionary spiral. An evolutionary historical diagnosis produces objective evaluation. Mindful that art's destiny, even where creative work defies heteronomous pressures by the vigor of its autonomy, hinges on the individual as well as the collective, the psychological as well as the social fate of humanity, such a diagnosis opens a vista to tomorrow by examining yesterday and today and duly values the detection of causality through conclusive interpretation.

Any analysis of the historical position and function of the work of art is simultaneously a judgment on its intrinsic value, since the arc of history, despite all the reversals, bends toward the expansion of freedom. Today it is truly imperative, as well as an axis of progressive energy, to be cognizant of the transformation painting has undergone from depicting exteriority, from "icon painting" and "nature painting," to poetry and the process whereby all art is being ushered into the realm of poetry. And the understanding that poetry, which springs from the same human sources as love, is moving like love toward the polestar of freedom warrants the prognosis that neither the overt nor covert impact of Štyrský's work will diminish for as long as poetry's supremacy continues to expand in the history of the human spirit, for he created an oeuvre that so distinctively and provocatively impacted the process of identifying painting with poetry. The power of his work will only grow in time, even if it were to be temporarily eclipsed only to be viewed later in its entirety as the harbinger of new discoveries. It will become the lodestar for new generations, who will judge and interpret it in their own ways, discovering for their own pursuits its focal point even in those moments that escape the gaze of today. Only when the poetic work displays its timeless relevance will its temporality also be palpable in full detail, its consonance, as an oeuvre, even if hermetically closed unto itself, with the zeitgeist of the era in which it was born. The full extent and impact of a poetry with the mission to actualize itself in life rather than being a reflection of life, that anticipates the possibilities of life rather than adapting itself to the realities of the world, can be fully understood only later. And yet such a poetry, perhaps like a rocket in the stratosphere, affirms rather than disproves the earthly, human, historical law of gravity while demonstrating the truism that the heights are reached only via the depths.

A painter who dies at the age of forty-three leaves with a secret still untold. The growing intensity of the real and the unalloyed surreality of lyrical fantasy in the final period of Štyrský's work suggests that its interrupted trajectory would lead from the materialization of the poetic imagination via the painting to an actualization of poetry in life, that the path taken by the poetic ideal, winged by primordial and universal human desire, from the depiction of fantastical objects to the fantastical juxtaposition of real objects is ultimately headed to the transformation of reality per the exigencies of desire, to the conversion of utopia into reality, to the transformation of life to align it with the ancient dream of humanity. Perceived in poetic pictures, this ancient dream is one of the vital sources of power that will transform life on earth into its image.

Karel Teige
Prague, 1948

DREAMS

1925–1940

Work birthed in the wellsprings of hypnagogic mental models, via faithful representations of dream objects and authentic dream records

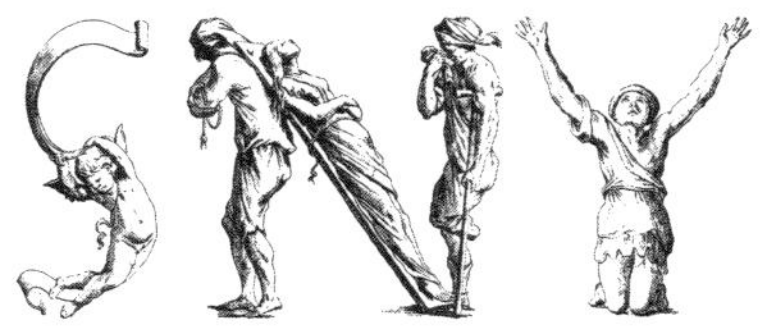

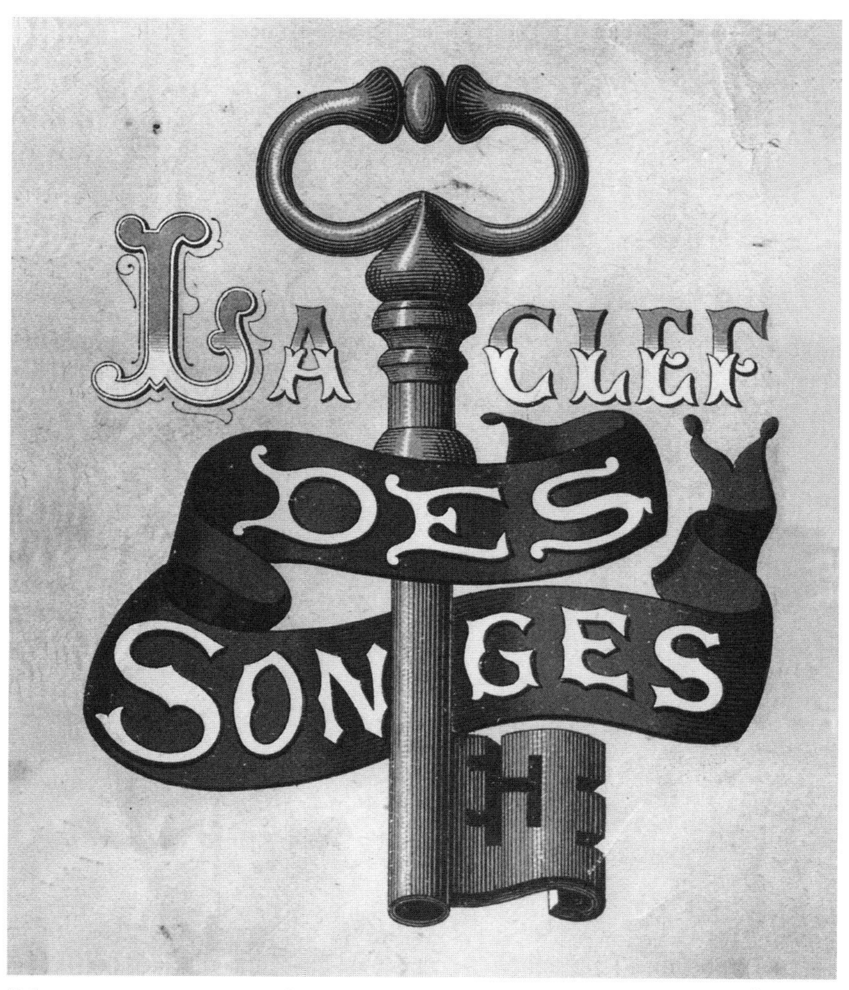

"The Key to Dreams," cover of a French dream book, undated, the final image in Štyrský's layout plan for *Dreams*.

Our dreams are a second life. I have never been able to penetrate without a shudder those ivory or horned gates which separate us from the invisible world.

Gérard de Nerval, *Aurélia*

Cézanne picked up a box in the hall and took me to his *motif*. It was two kilometers away with a view over a valley at the foot of Sainte-Victoire, the rugged mountain he continually painted in watercolor and in oils and which filled him with great admiration.

Emile Bernard, *Memories of Paul Cézanne*

I am also going to my *motif*, into my dreams.

Jindřich Štyrský

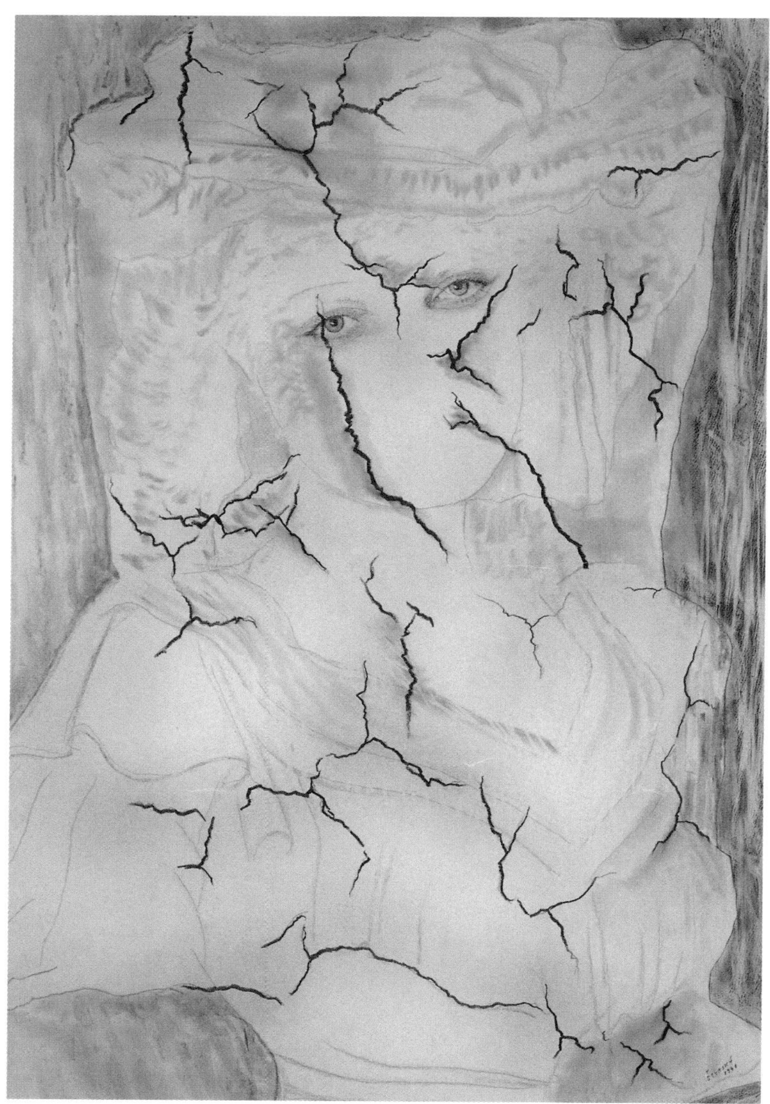

Portrait of My Sister Marie, 1941, charcoal on paper

As a young child I saw in the color supplement of a magazine the image of a woman's head, exquisite with golden hair, whose pale hue will always suggest azure to me. Her lips, red with lipstick, looked like a moist chasm, though silent, slightly parted, and mute. Eyes of violet — in them pride, sin, and weakness — blazed in a pallid face. The head was perverse, yet full of compassion, damned, yet full of kindness. It was the head of Medusa, the whole of it in a pool of blood. Blood streamed from its neck, and its hair was a cluster of vipers, erect, ready to penetrate the woman through her mouth, nose, and ears. I gave little mind to who had painted the picture, thus the artist's name has been effaced from my memory, but the horror depicted there has never left me. A ghastly horror, an alluring horror. Head of Medusa. It kept recurring in my dreams. I tried to place this head on those closest to me at that time : my mother and sister. The head was a perfect fit on my sister. So I was madly in love with her. In the depths of my memories of my sister lies the memory of her death. Her bare legs, strained by spasm, readying for the journey to the underworld. Spurs were strapped to her feet. Those long, distrustful, perfidious legs with the ankles of Beardsley's women and calves of chiseled flesh. My sister was delirious, like the delirium of a water plant in moonlight. She blossomed in agony like a succulent medium in a trance, like a large nocturnal flower. I regret that I didn't get to know her fragrance. When remembering today, this woman appears to me like a foal sleeping in an alpine wilderness. She certainly knew the many ways of love. Thus I instinctively created my CHIMERA, my PHANTOM OBJECT, on which I am fixated and to which I dedicate this work.

J.Š.
Prague, May 1941

I

Dreams of the Snake and the Miraculous Pear

(1925–30)

When dozing off and when dreaming, I was regularly haunted by a slit-open snake, eviscerated, bereft of its guts. Sometimes it was a snake without an end — like chain-link — sometimes a snake without a head. I often awoke in terror as it was coiled around my neck. Though strangling me, I did not find its touch revolting, it felt good. The snake appeared in a variety of scenes, sometimes accompanied by a pear. I called it *The Miraculous Pear*. I'm convinced these two phenomena are connected.

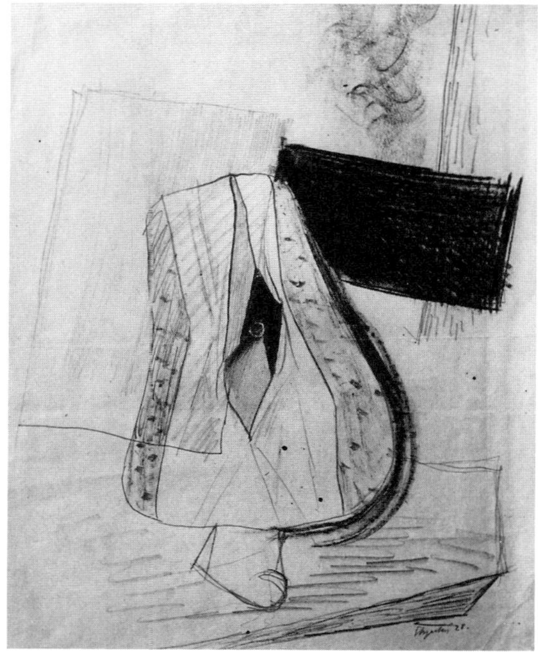

The Miraculous Pear, 1928, pencil and pastel on paper

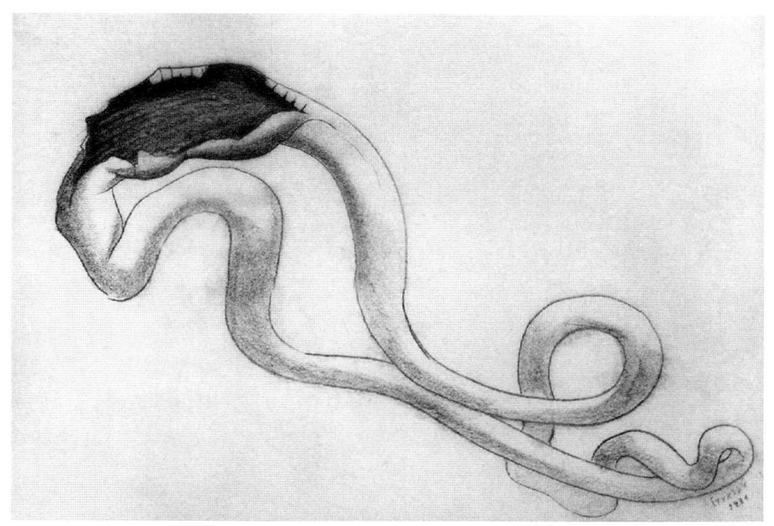

Infinite Snake, 1931, pencil and pastel on paper

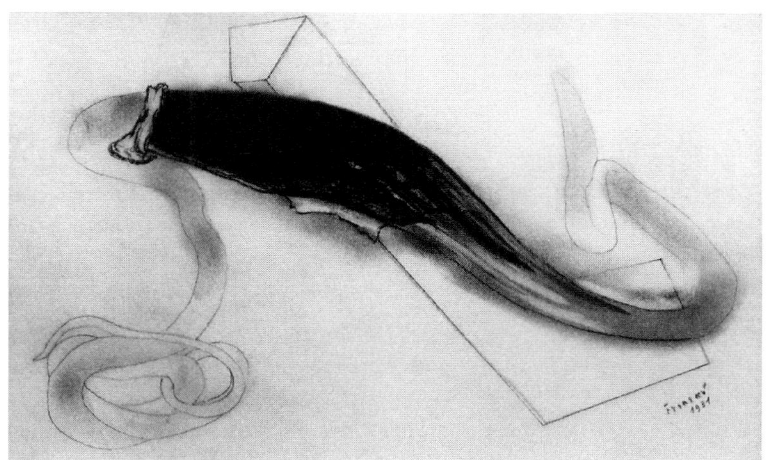

Gutted Snake, 1931, pencil and pastel on paper

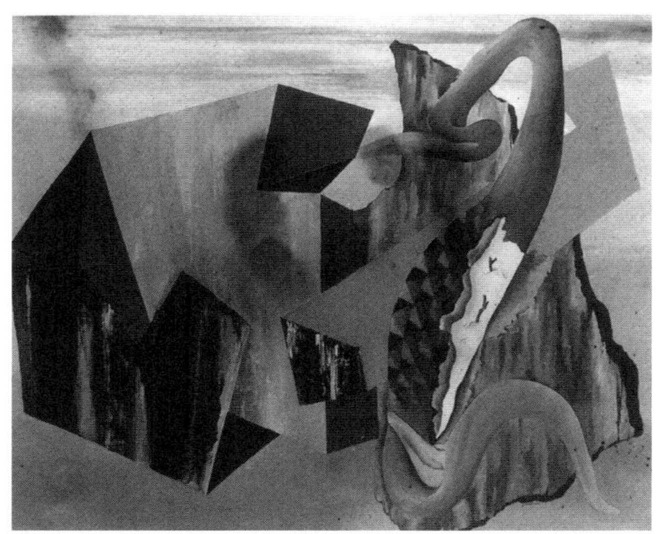

On the Beach, 1931, oil on canvas (lost)

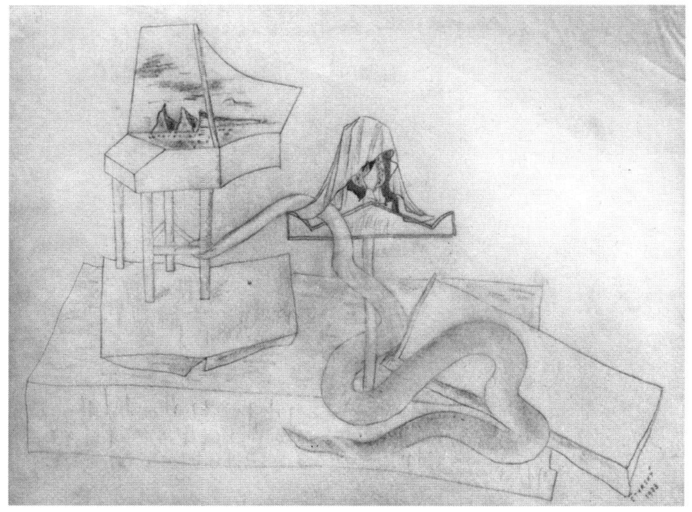

The Miraculous Pear with Snake, 1933, pencil and pastel on paper

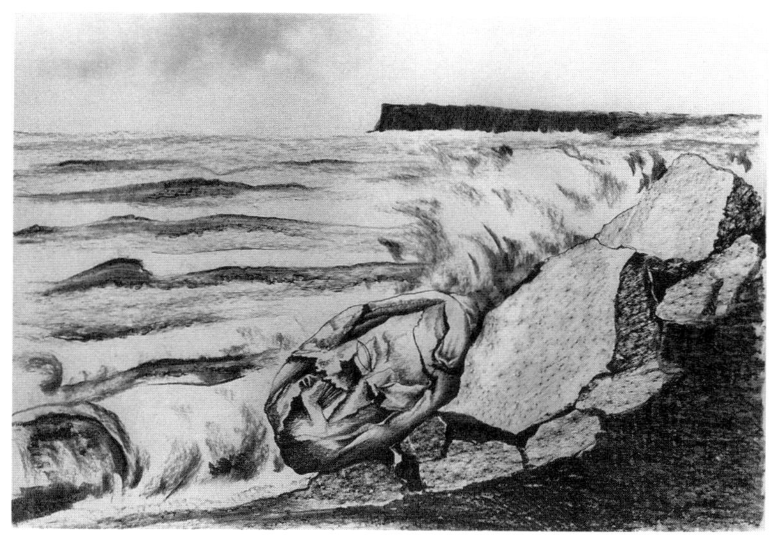

Apocalypse I, 1929, pencil and frottage on paper

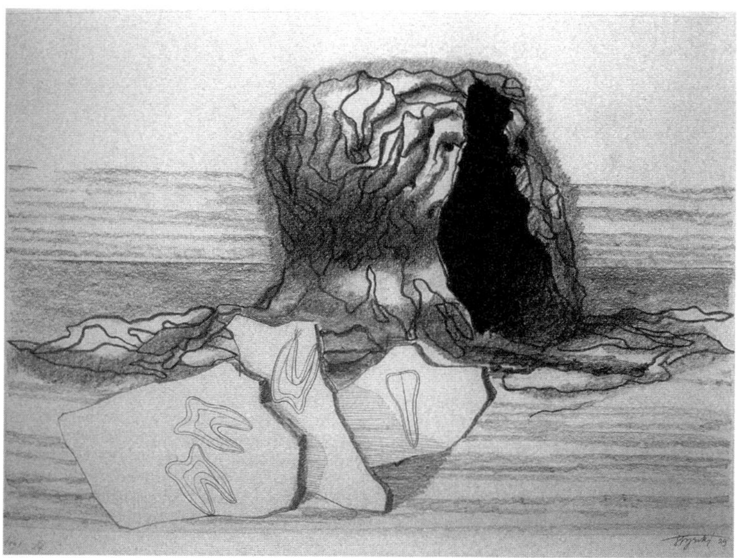

Apocalypse II, 1929, pencil and frottage on paper

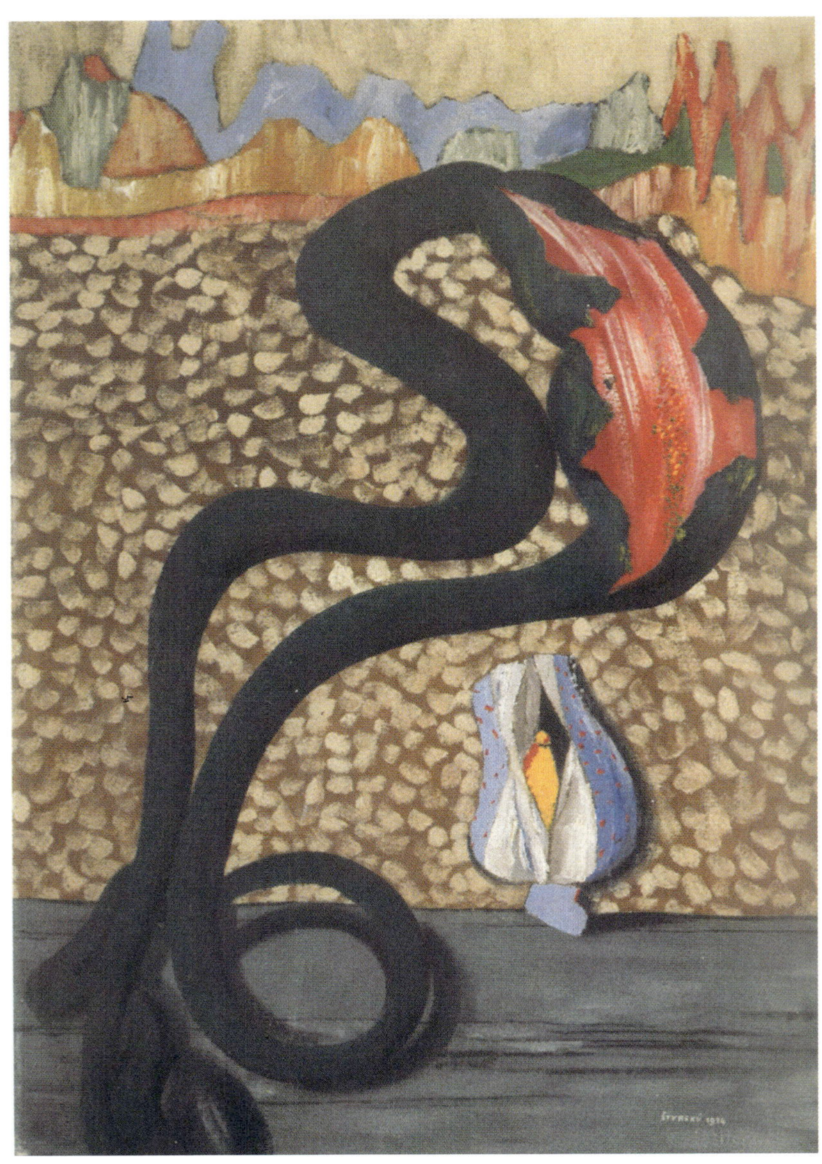

Hermaphrodite, 1934, oil on canvas

II

Dreams of Two Small Snakes

(1934)

The pear later vanished, and rather than a single snake there were two small snakes, dancing before me, sometimes kissing. One was green and the other red. Then the two small snakes vanished from my sleep.

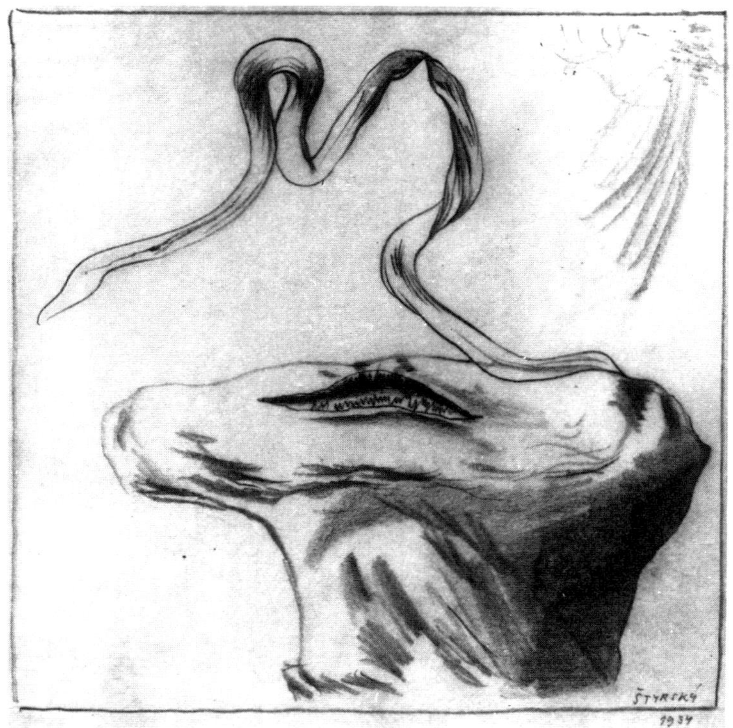

Two Small Snakes, 1934, pencil on paper

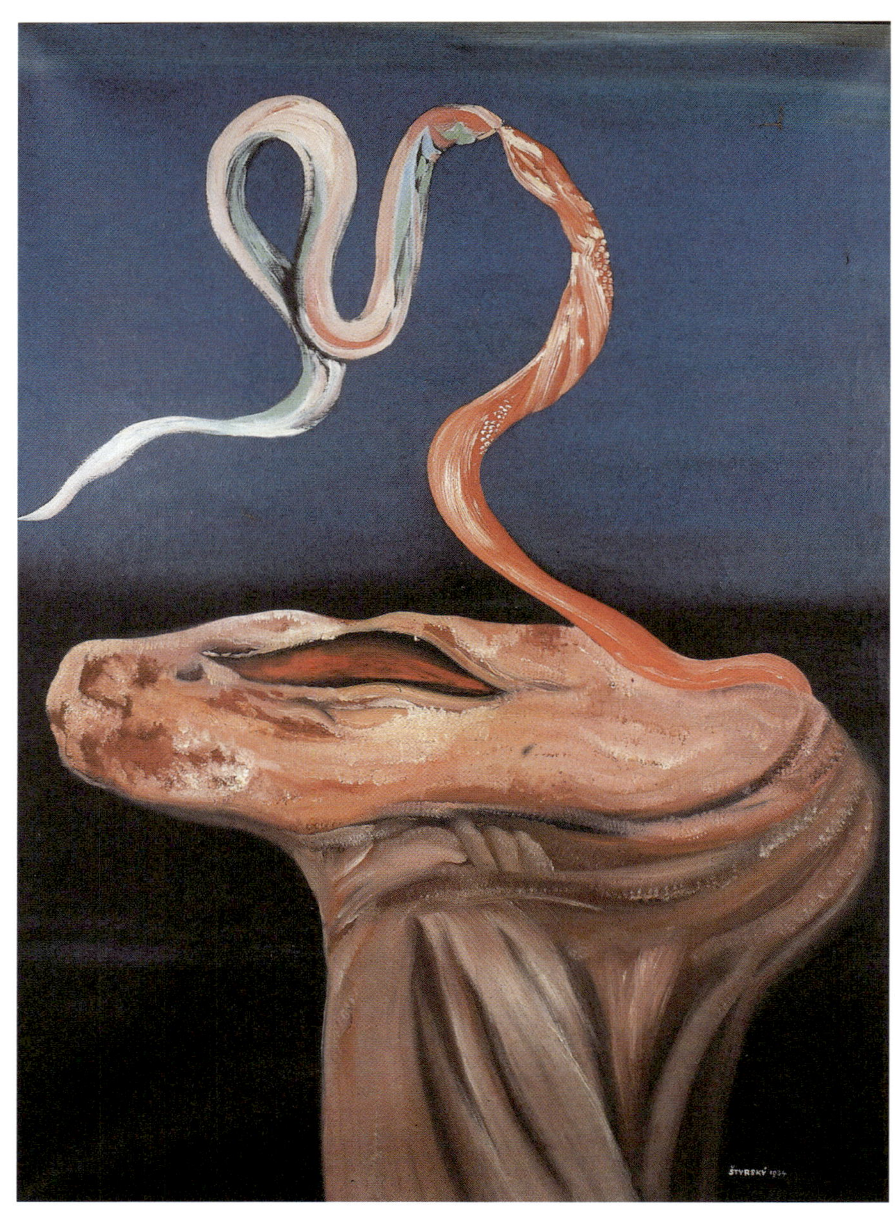

Man Cephalopod, 1934, oil on canvas

III

Dream of Snakes

(1940)

In 1940, the snakes appeared once again in different form. I have kept the first sketch of this dream :

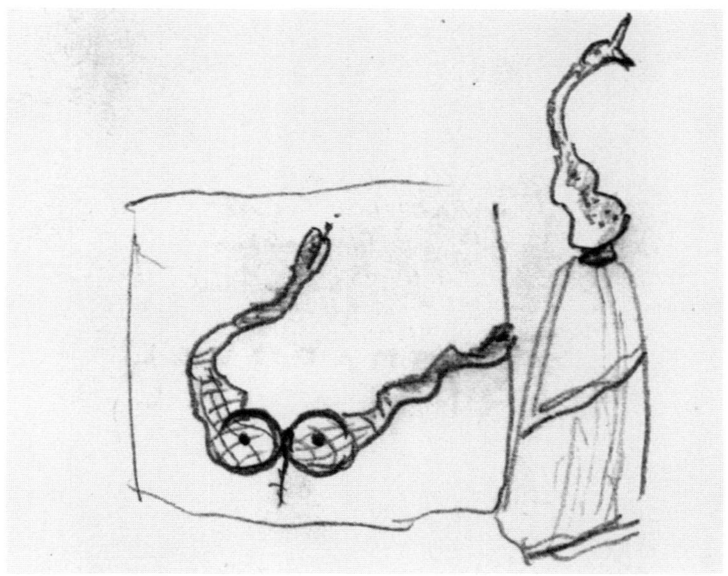

Dream Sketch, 1940, pencil on paper

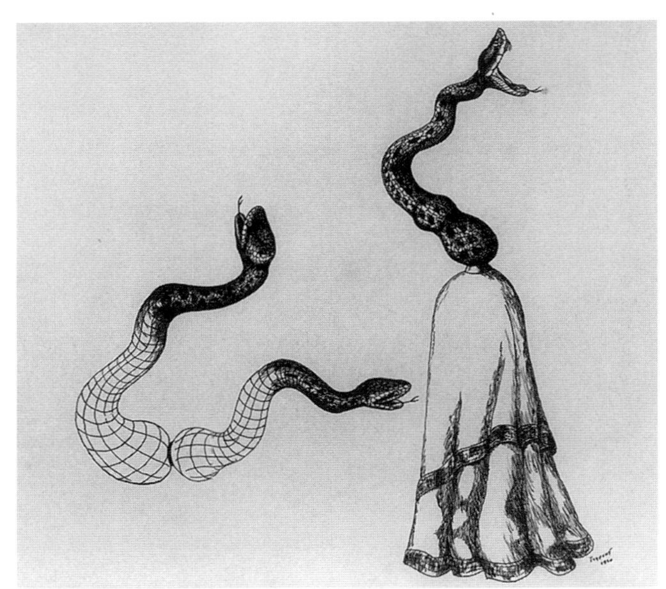

Dream of Snakes I, 1940, pen and ink on paper

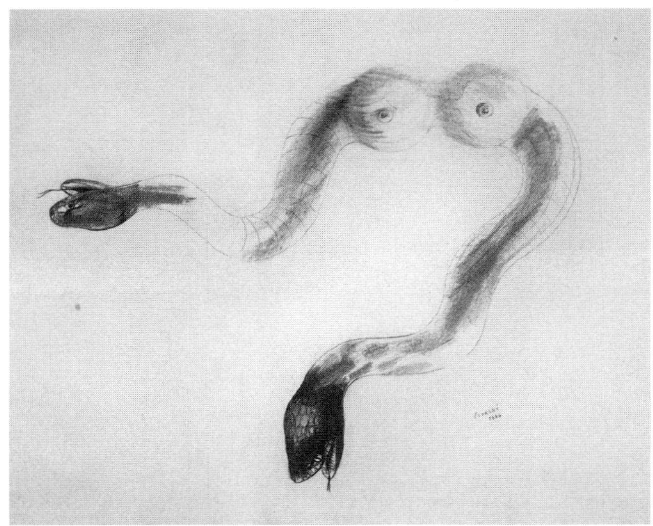

Dream of Snakes II, 1940, pencil on paper

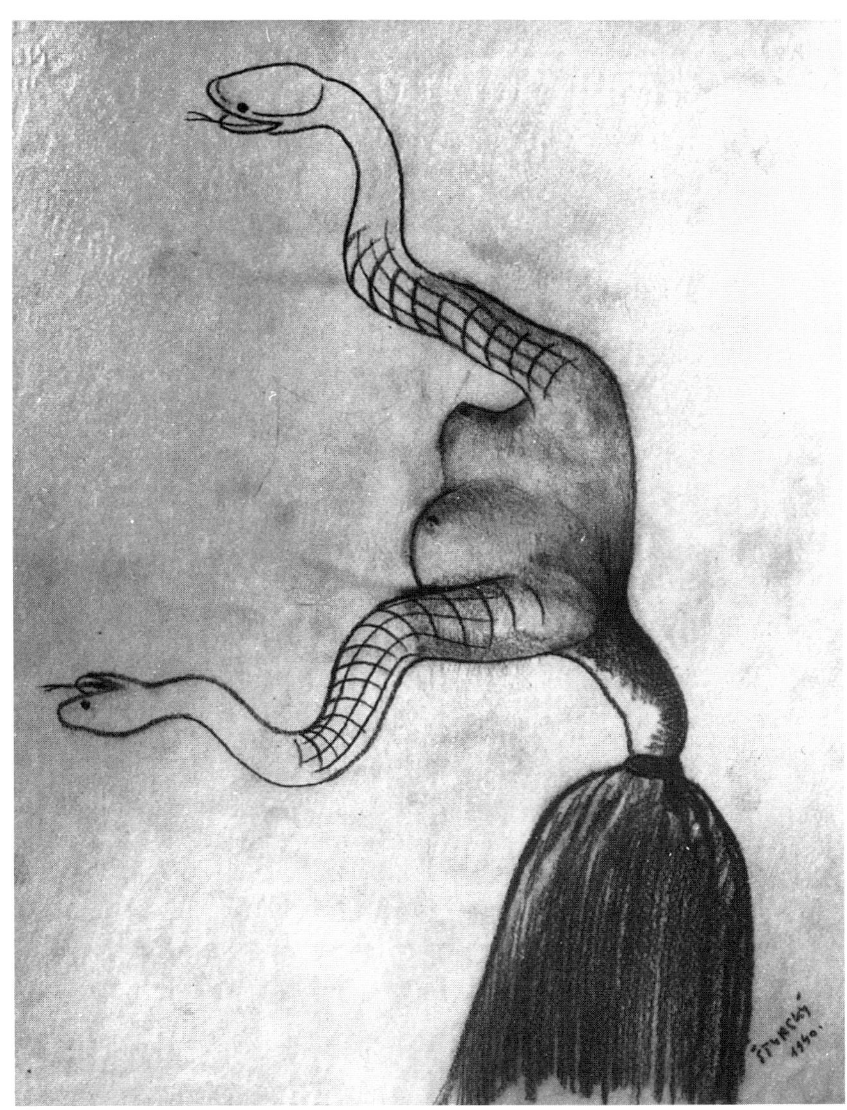

Dream of Snakes III, 1940, pencil on paper

IV

Dream of the Marten

(1925)

In the dream I was walking along a headland. The rocks here formed an odd sort of pass. I wandered until I reached a large modern villa with a terrace and gazebo draped in grapevine. In the moonlight it looked to me like backstage at the Paris Opera. Wanting to spend the night in the gazebo, I climbed over the wall. My drowsing was disturbed by shutters opening on the first floor, which emitted a light that was engulfed by the crown of a leafy palm. A woman leaned out the window. I was unable to determine her age since she appeared to me as a silhouette. Her hair struck me as peculiar as it was done up in an outmoded bun. Then I saw her hair was *white*, and as she moved I could see the glitter of pearls sewn onto ribbons plaited into it. The woman leaned out the window and quietly called out : "I'll redeem the box when the night's over." From the top of the palm above me I suddenly heard the melody of a tired ditty. When I looked to see who was singing, I saw a giant orangutan playing a fiddle. He had a ruby red box hanging from a strap with an odd handle in the shape of a child's hand. On the branch of a tree standing near the palm sat a large marten, its head erect as if an old illustration in a natural history book, as if fascinated by the singing. It had been flayed, and the skin and hairs on its neck gave way to raw flesh, which was larded with bacon fat like a hare ready for roasting.

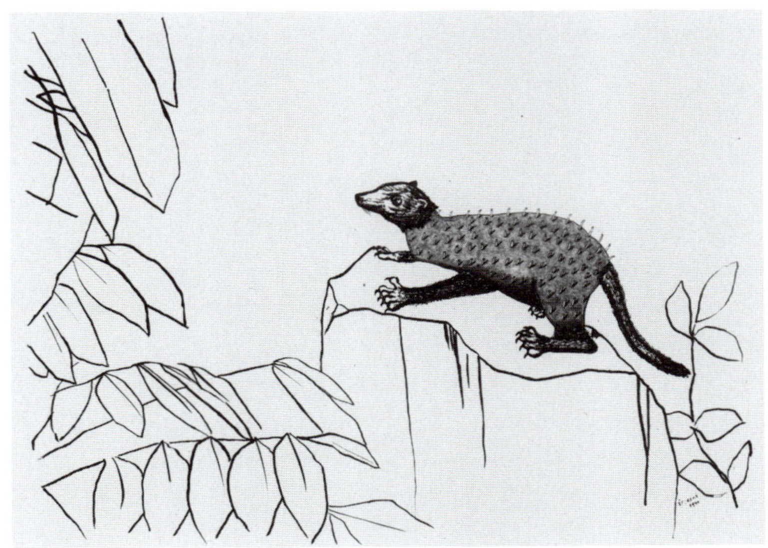

Dream of the Marten I, 1940, India ink and pastel on paper

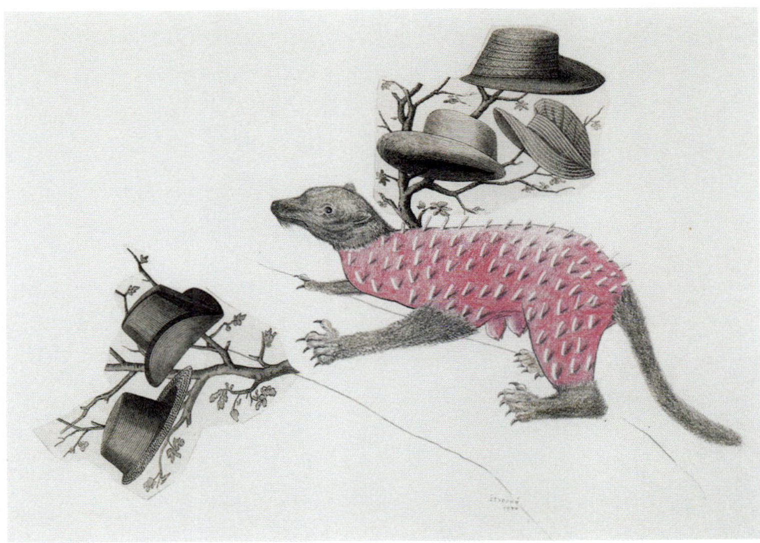

Dream of the Marten II, 1940, pencil, pastel, and collage on paper

V

Dream of Emilie

(NIGHT OF JULY 5–6, 1926)

I am in my parents' garden. In front of the house and its small steps is a tiny enclosed garden of currants. The fruit trees here are in the exact same place as they are in reality. But I am surprised to find a baroque gate giving onto a vast park and an *underground passage*, everywhere cascades of water, terracotta gnomes, garden castles, Chinese lanterns, and the ground strewn with salami skins and cheese wrappings. White tables, set as in a garden café, stand between the trees. I am aware that all these things do not actually belong here. I am with Emilie. Suddenly she's not with me, and I'm watching C. bathe in our fishpond, which is situated in an unfamiliar landscape. It seems as if he's been there since yesterday. It's noon, but he keeps shouting that it's only *10 a.m.* Once more I'm in the garden, where a strange auto driving through the air squirms its way between the trees. Its inventor, a little gray man, is talking. On a path through the meadow I kiss his hand, which he accepts with an odd sort of satisfaction. Then I am accompanying Emilie and feel as though I abandoned her 20 years ago. She is telling me about the parties she is hosting today, tomorrow, and the day after. We kiss on the steps, and she unbuttons my pants, wanting to show her love for me in every way possible. All of a sudden Father is shouting at me that he's going to shoot me with a No. 10 revolver.

VI

Second Dream of Emilie

(OCTOBER 2, 1926)

I am about 8–10 years old, and Emilie and I are playing with dolls in the garden at Čermná. The dolls are broken : headless, legless, only having SOMETHING like a head.* I am at the spot where a very special type of plum tree grew in my childhood and later withered. It is summer, and the entire garden is covered in a high, dense, luxuriant grass that is growing everywhere the earth is damp. The area under the plum tree has been cut. No one can see us. Overripe plums have fallen and lay scattered on the ground. Workers are erecting a fence around the garden. I remark that 4 x 35 posts will be needed. We run through the high grass toward the posts. Deep holes have already been dug along the road. My pockets are full of assorted bits of broken coffee mugs, plates, pitchers bearing painted flowers, ornaments, pieces of a landscape, pieces of a face, shards of drinking glasses with engraved roses, etc. I throw all of it into the holes, though I regret doing so, yet tell Emilie it has to be done to make the fence sturdy. Emilie also wants to contribute, so she unwraps her cone of candy and tosses green menthol lozenges into the holes. Then we sit down by the hole into which we've thrown all the broken dolls and out of nowhere a post is standing there, alternately dancing in the hole like a pestle in a mortar and laboriously moving up and down like a paper pulper.

I have recorded this *important* dream for the vivid impression that stayed with me upon waking : I make love like a child.

* *Graveyard of Dolls,* author's note, 1941.

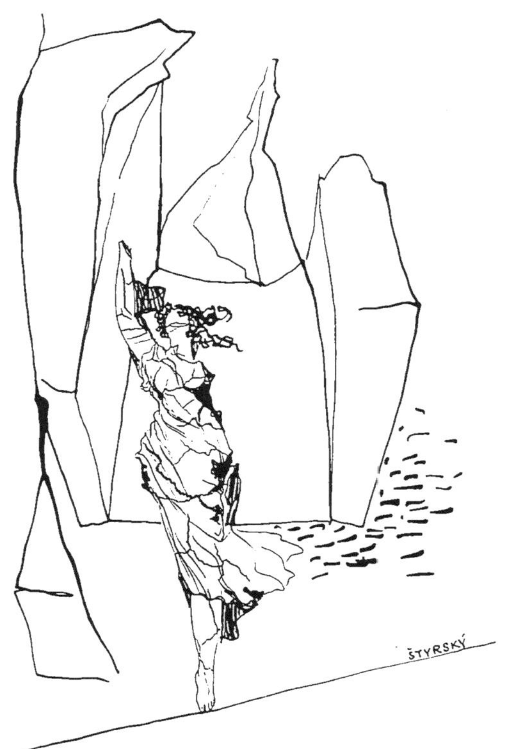

Eurydice, 1930, pen and ink on paper

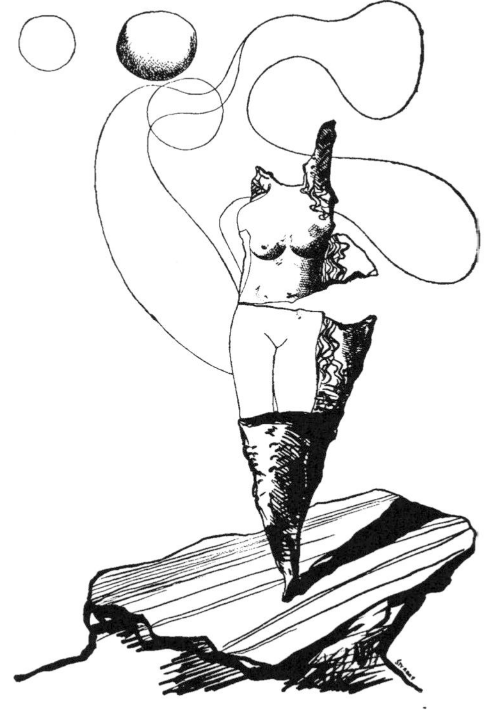

Quiet I, 1932, pen and ink on paper

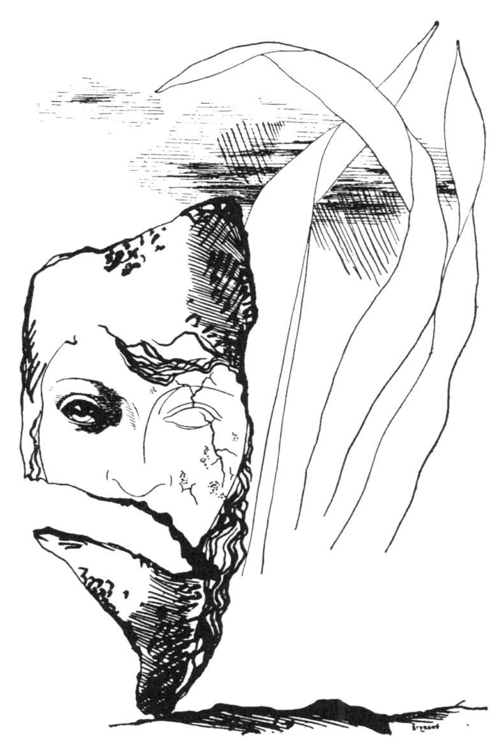

Quiet II, 1932, pen and ink on paper

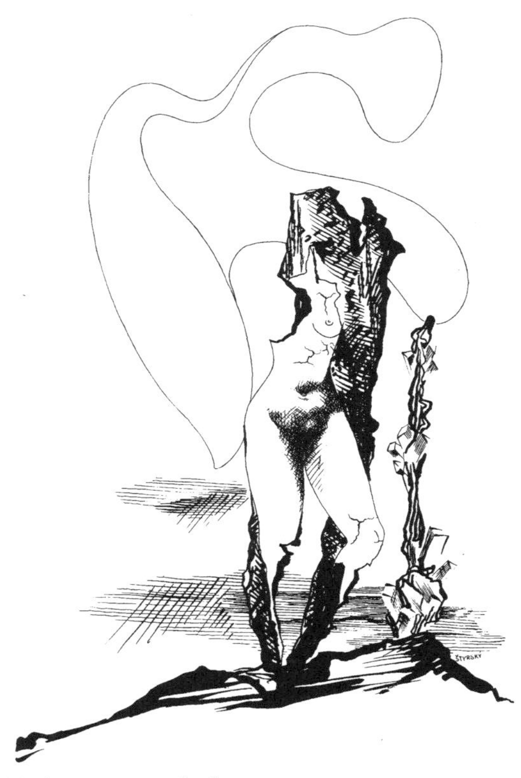

Torso, 1934, pen and ink on paper

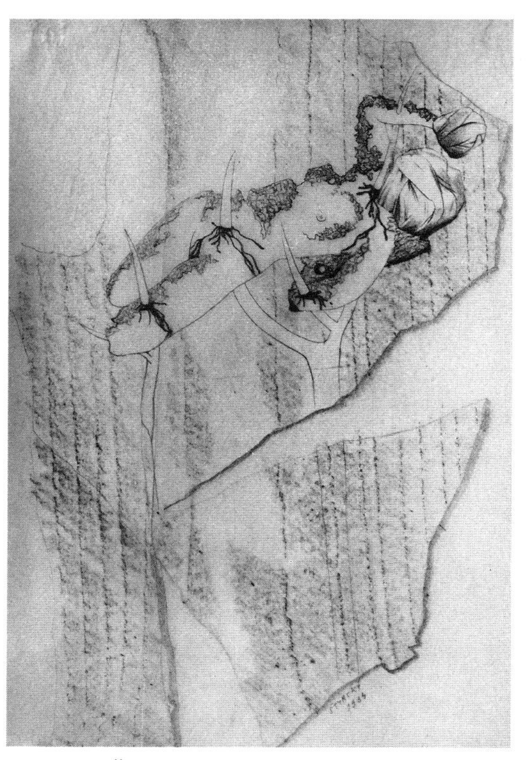

Sketch for *Čerchov* I, 1934, pencil on paper

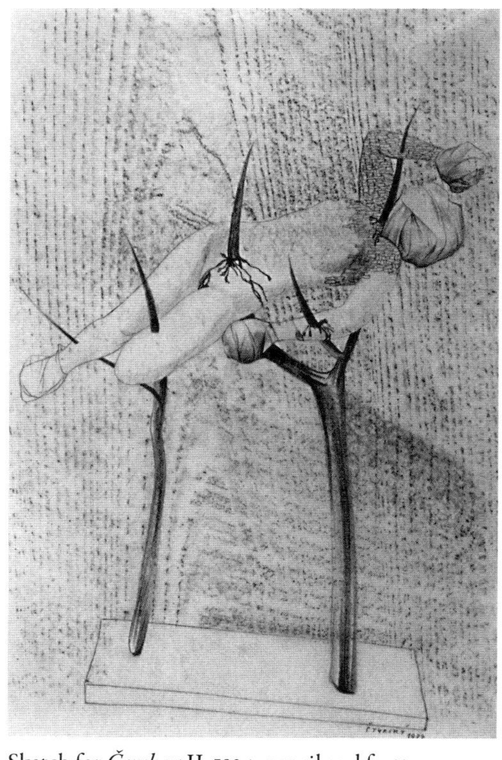

Sketch for *Čerchov* II, 1934, pencil and frottage on pape

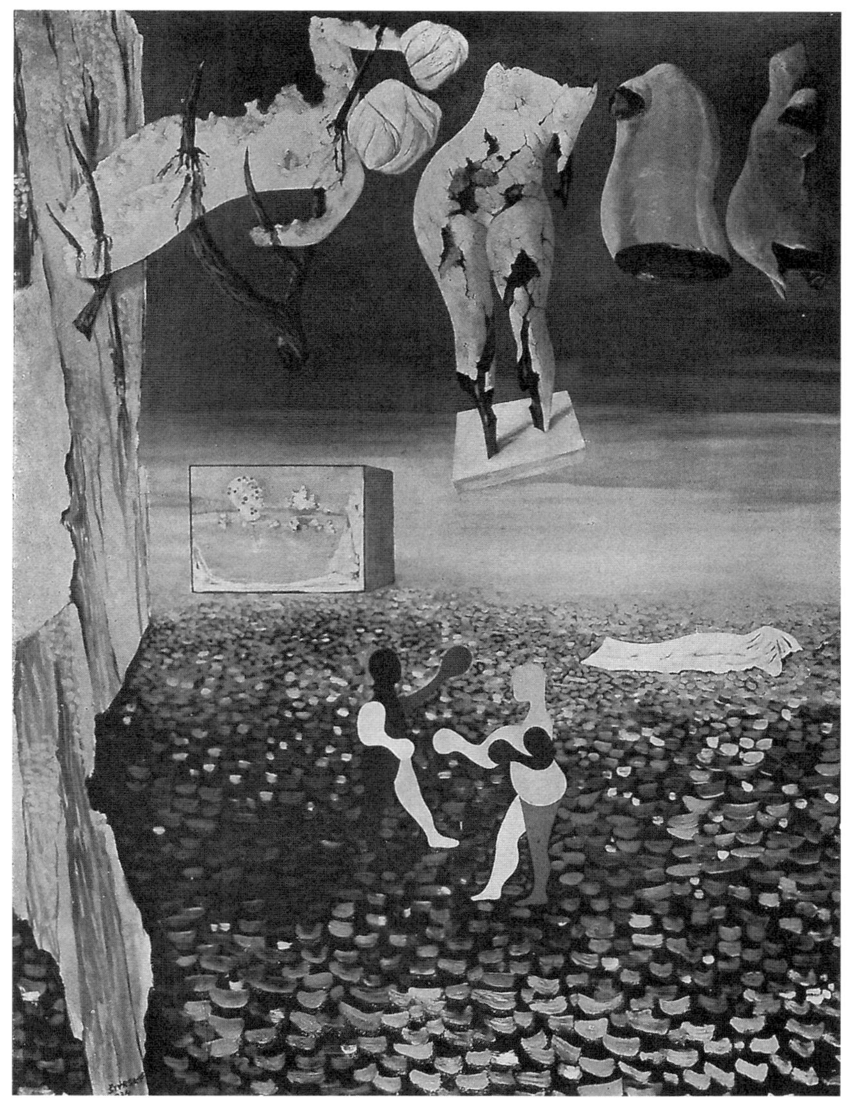

Čerchov, 1934, oil on canvas (lost)

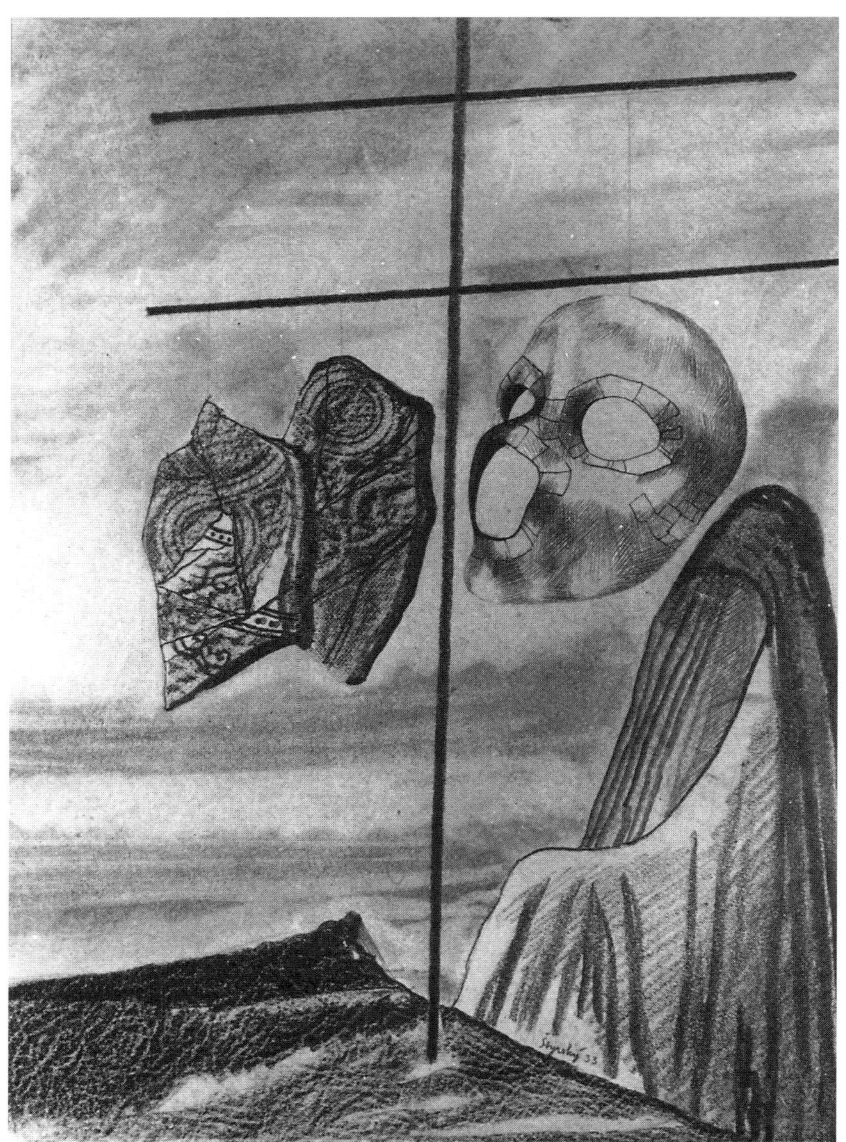

Untitled, 1933, pencil and frottage on paper

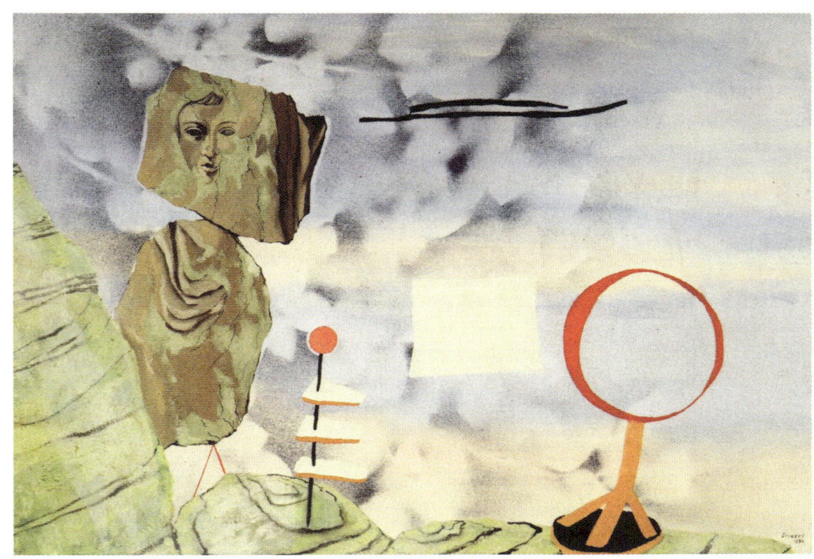

Untitled, 1932, oil on canvas

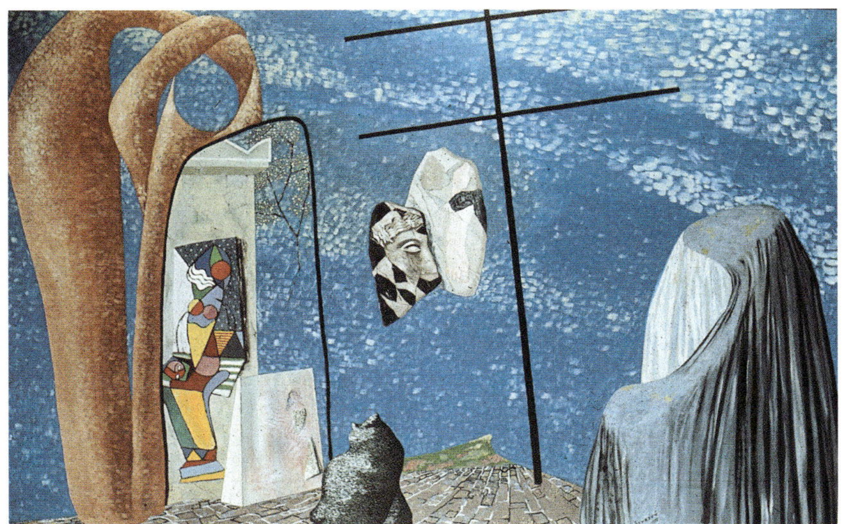

From My Diary, 1933, oil on canvas

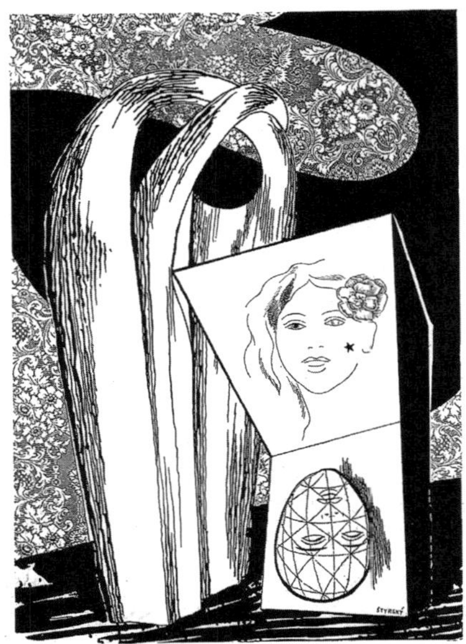

From My Diary, 1933, India ink and collage on paper

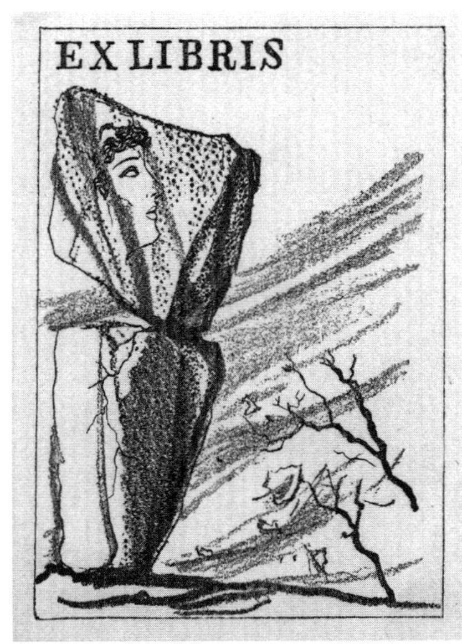

Ex libris, 1932, colored pencil on paper

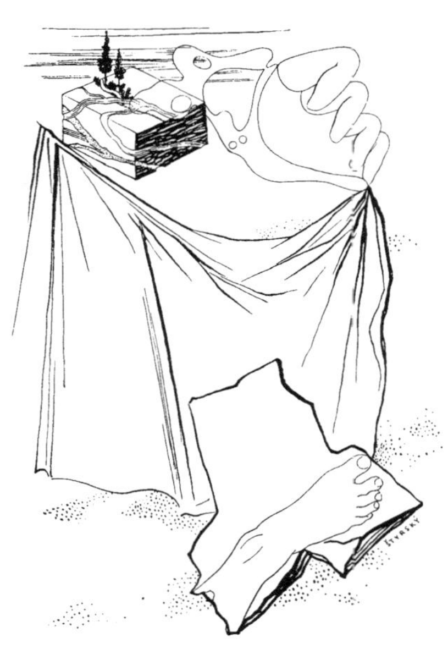

Landscape with Foot, 1933, pen and ink on paper

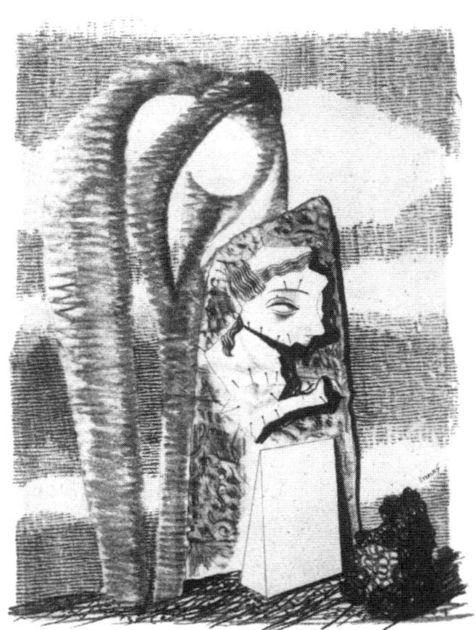

Sketch to *From My Diary,* 1933, pencil on paper

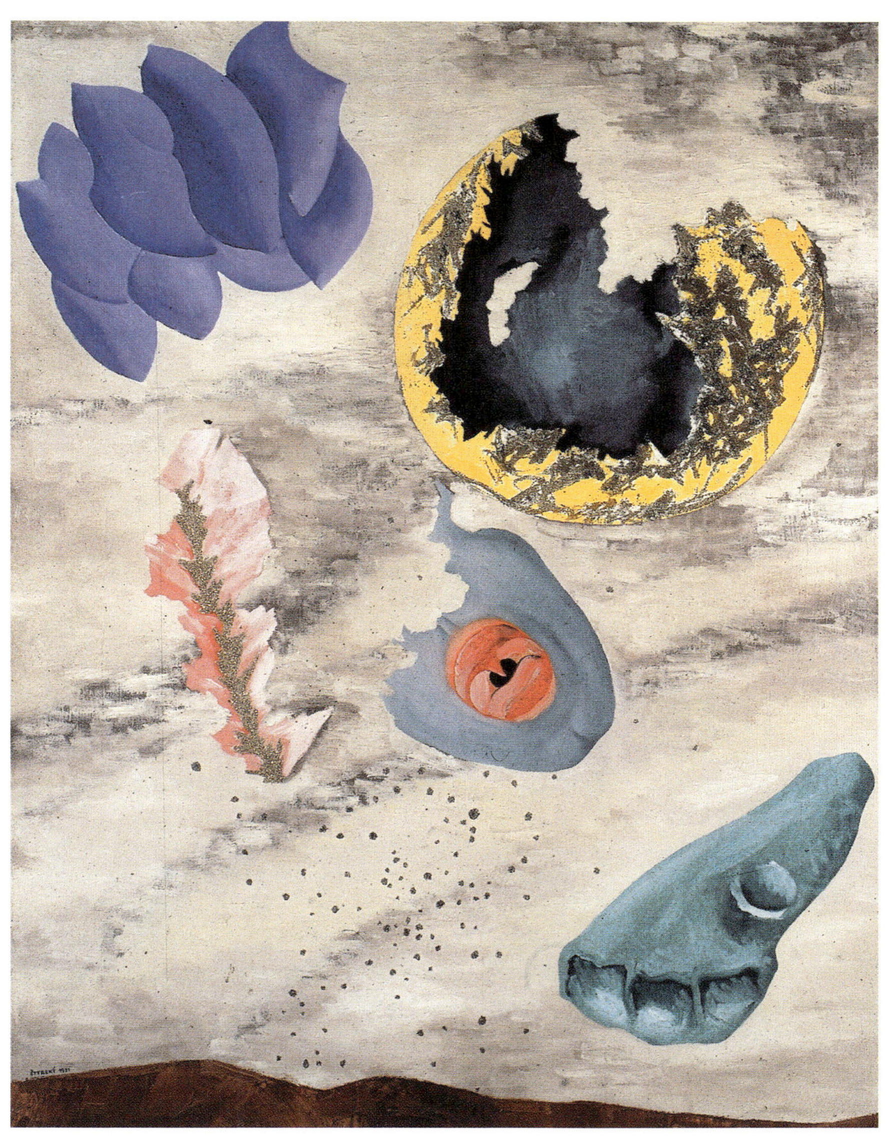

Palmetto, 1931, oil on canvas

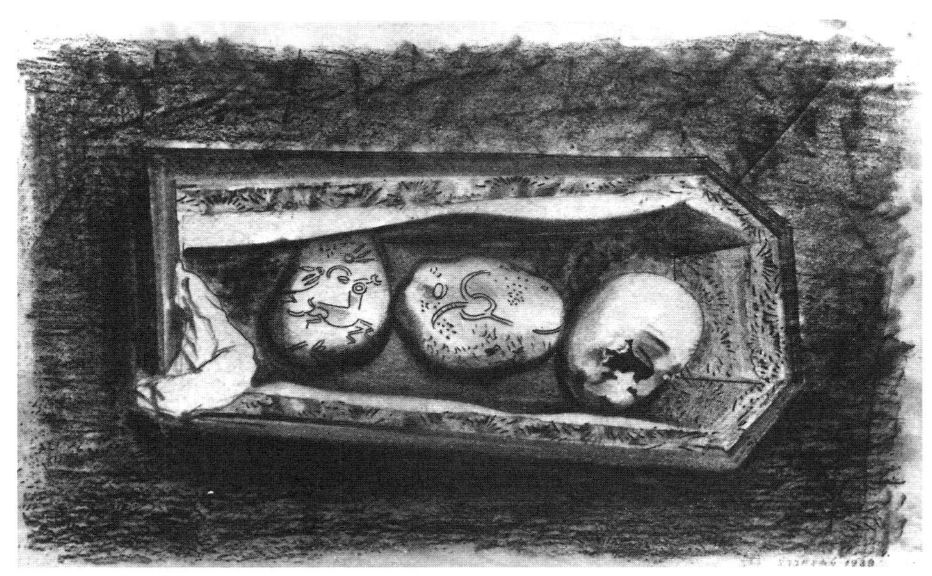

Buried Stones, 1939, pencil and frottage on paper

Sketch for a Tombstone, 1934, pencil on paper

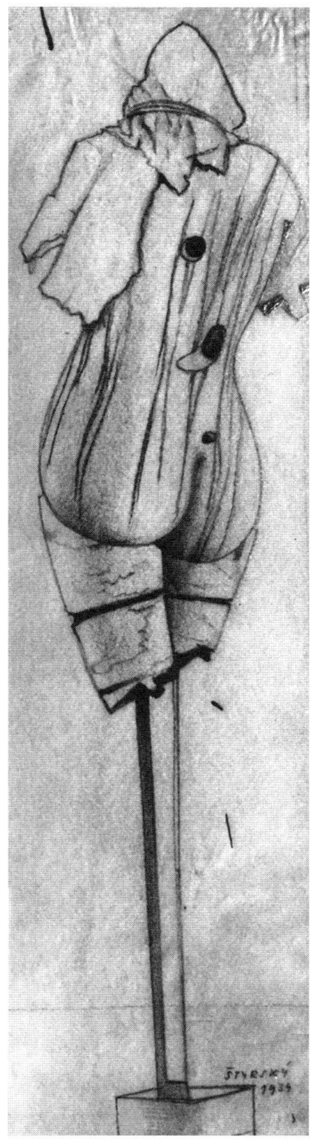

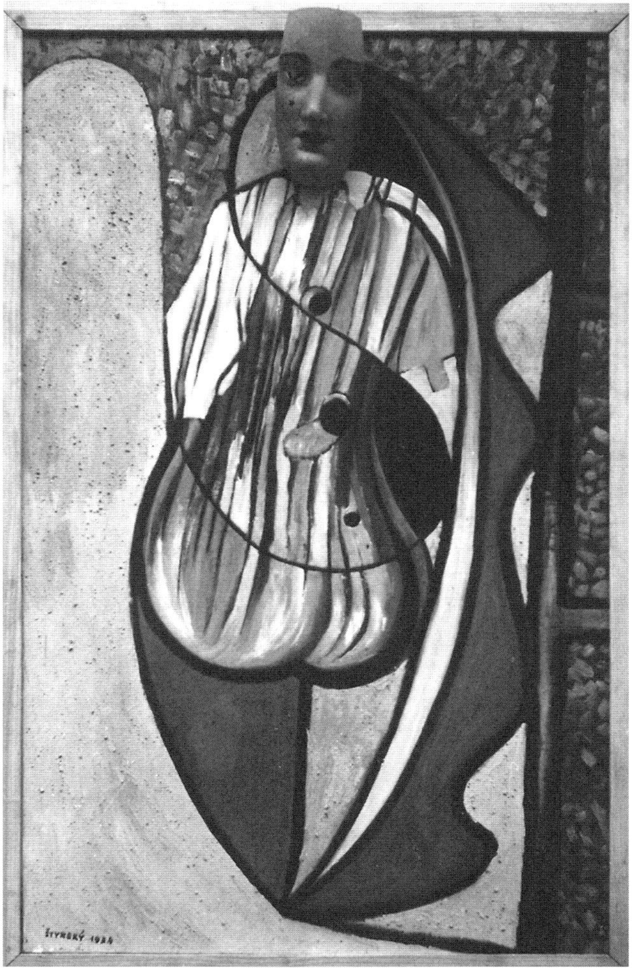

Tombstone, 1934, oil on canvas with affixed mask

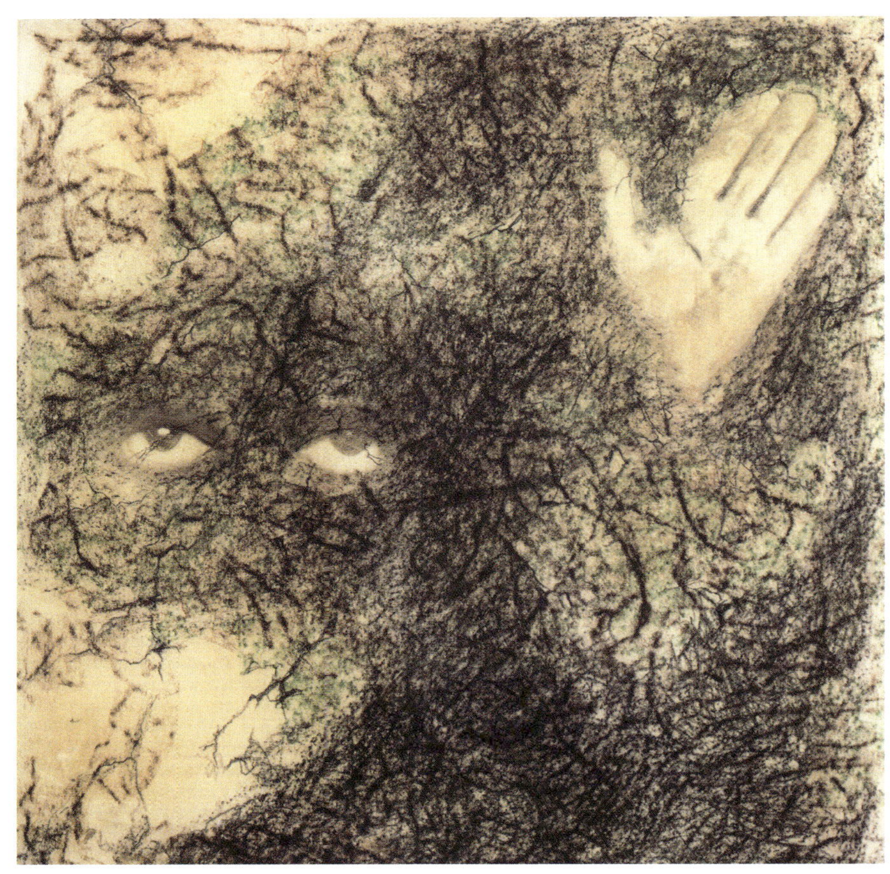

The Omnipresent Eye, 1936, pencil and pastel on paper

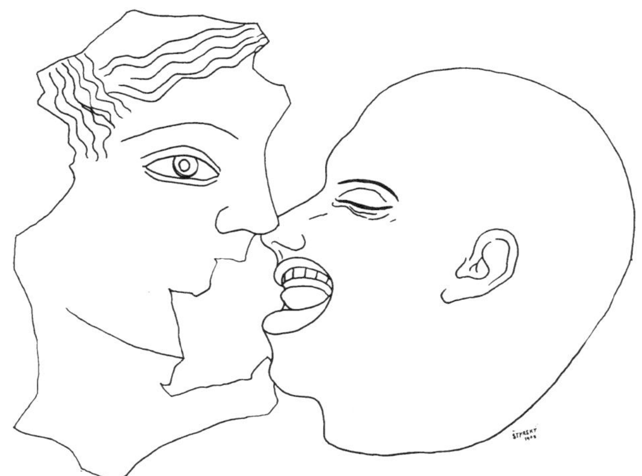

Kiss, 1939, pen and ink on paper

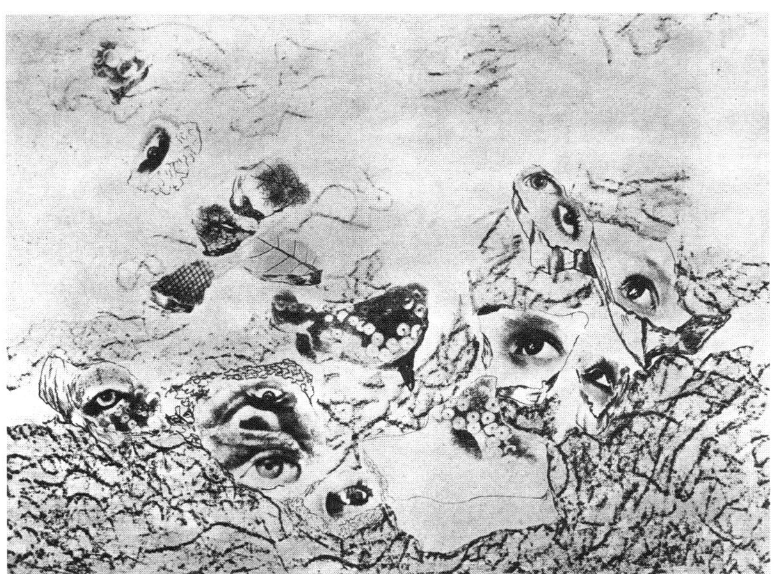

The Omnipresent Eye IV, 1936, charcoal and frottage on paper

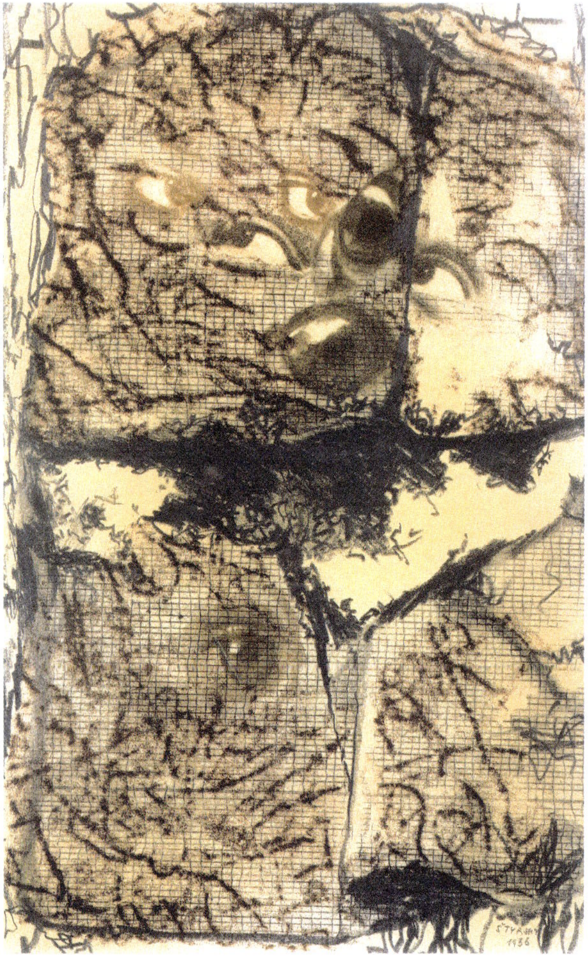

The Omnipresent Eye III, 1936, charcoal, ruddle, pastel and lithography on paper

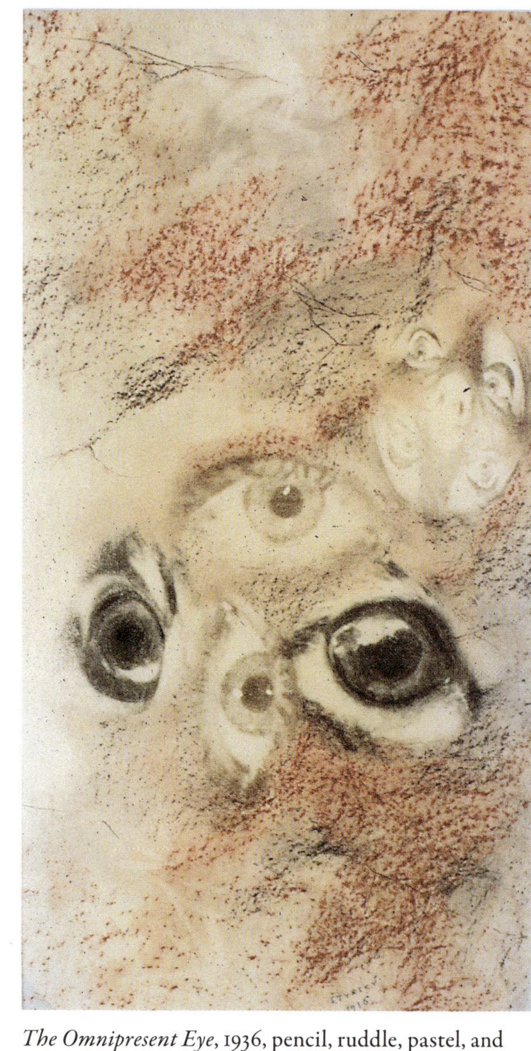

The Omnipresent Eye, 1936, pencil, ruddle, pastel, and frottage on paper

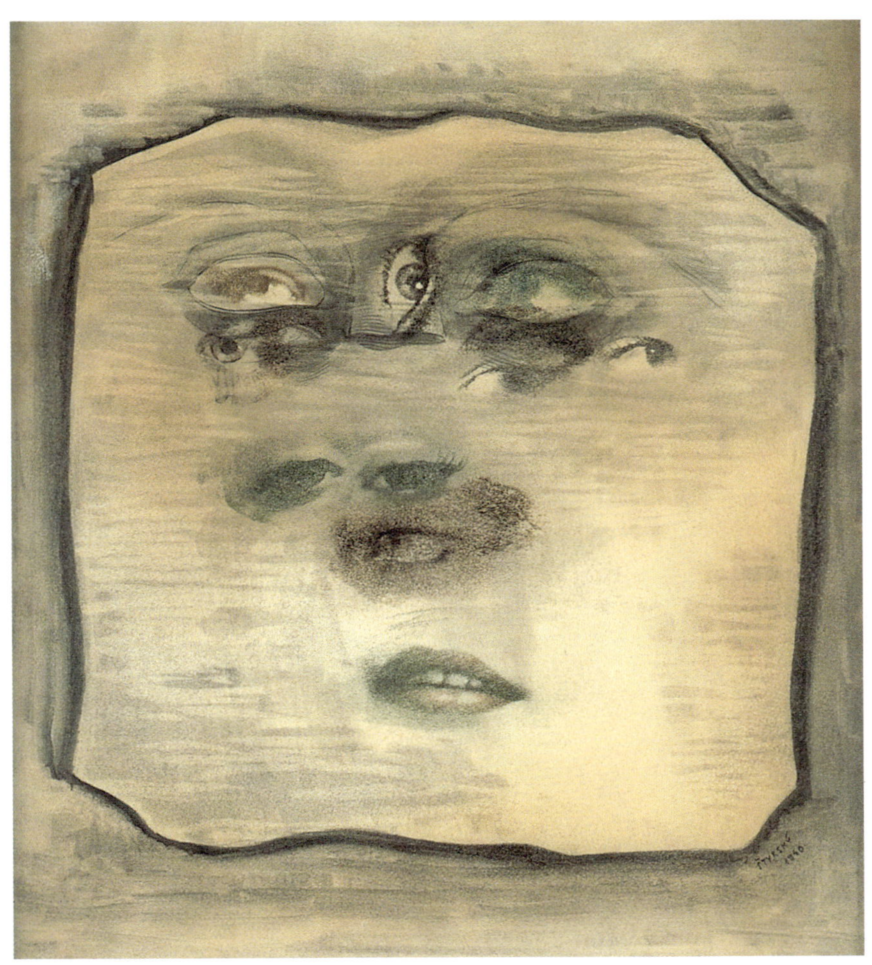

The Omnipresent Eye XVI, 1940, pencil and pastel on paper

VII

Dream of Vítězslav Nezval

(FEBRUARY 15, 1927)

. . . I'm telling Mother and Father about something that happened to me in Paris. Father has to take a business trip to Berlin — — — I'm looking for someone (I don't want to say it's Toyen) in Les Halles. I come to a house, open the door — — narrow — — I enter the parlor — — no one — — first floor, no one — — — darkness — — I go upstairs, no one — — I cough — — I call out "hello" — — no one — — when I'm on the third floor I'm overcome with terror and fly downstairs — — no one — — A blank — — — — I don't know — — — — — in front of the house is a small square (the Moor Café), flagstones, about which I say : large as a room. Nezval's lying in a chest, a coffin — — Backing up (I'm leaving the house with someone) a man says : he was a fat one, he liked his booze — — Nezval is lying in the small coffin, his legs tucked up, someone takes a leg and breaks it off, and then the other, and lays them down — — — shoe soles in his armpits — — — — — Teige somehow appears — — — before that someone, evidently the man I had left the house with, was rifling through Nezval's pants pockets, but it isn't there; he finds it in his wallet. Nezval seems alive, still lying there, and his hands refuse to give up the wallet. Teige says we need to take it from him, that he shouldn't be buried with money. At this point I wake up.

Papež české literatury

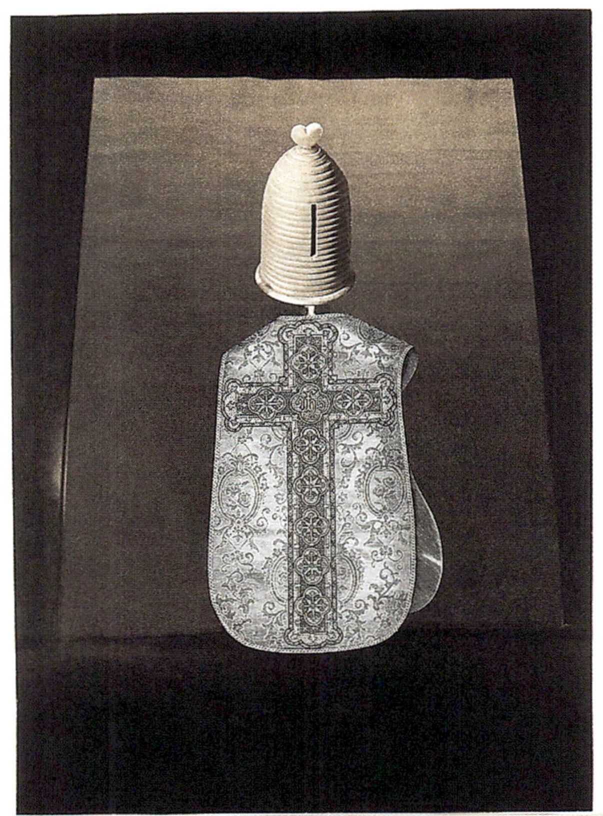

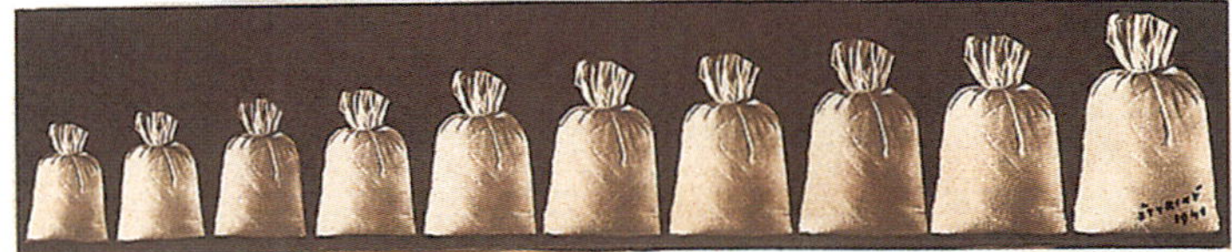

The Pope of Czech Literature, 1941, collage on paper

VIII

Dream of the Tiny Alabaster Hand

(MAY 25, 1928)

. . . we're running from the garden. Mrs. Jansová is with us. It is evening. Someone is pursuing us. We're in a room and I want to quickly close the windows. I shout at the others to run to the next room and close those windows. I am using both hands to remove the rods that are fastened to the windows to keep the wind from blowing them shut, when I see a delicate white hand slide out from the bushes growing right next to the house and hold back the left window sash, preventing my closing it. Then I run to the other window and shut it easily. From the next room they announce that all the windows are closed. I breathe a sigh of relief and tell Emilie : This was BEYOND DOUBT the tiny alabaster hand.

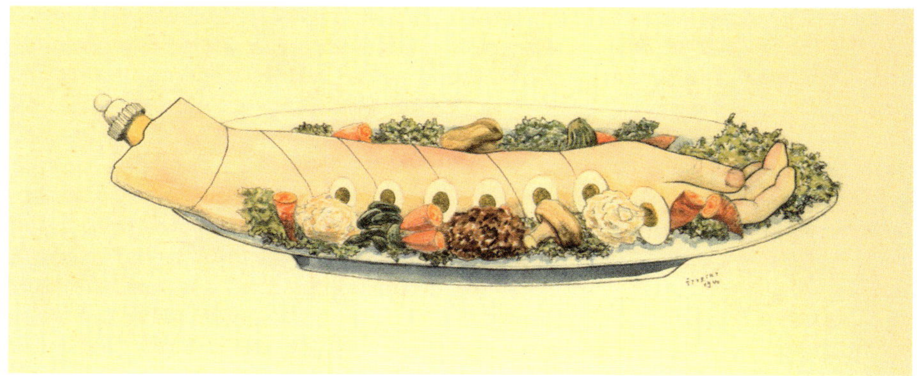

Bon appétit, 1940, pencil and watercolor on paper

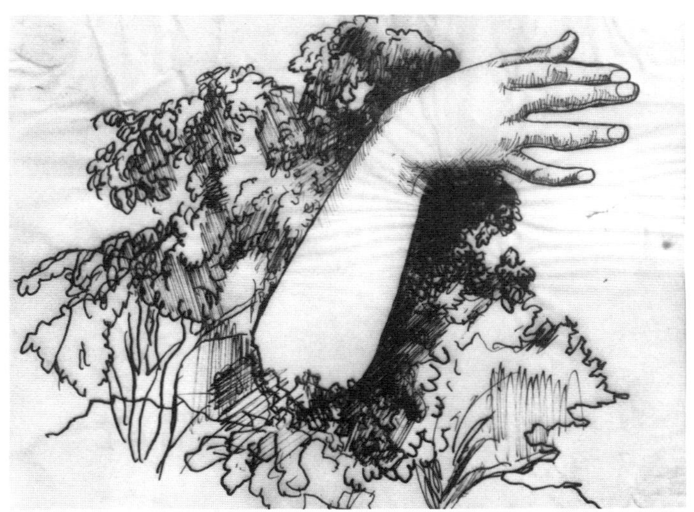

Dream Record, 1940, pen and ink on paper

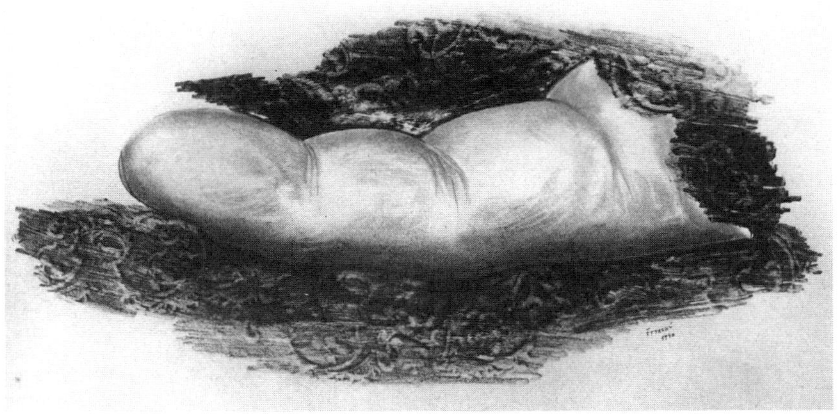

The Tiny Alabaster Hand, 1940, pencil, ruddle, and frottage on paper

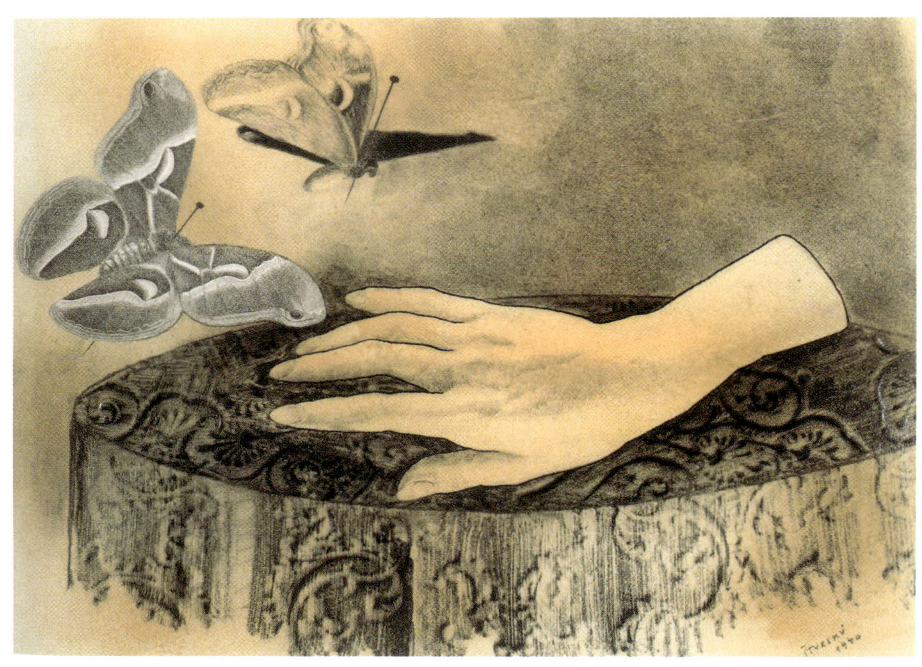

The Tiny Alabaster Hand, 1940, pencil, collage, and frottage on paper

IX

Dream of the Gypsy Woman

(3 A.M., APRIL 23, 1929)

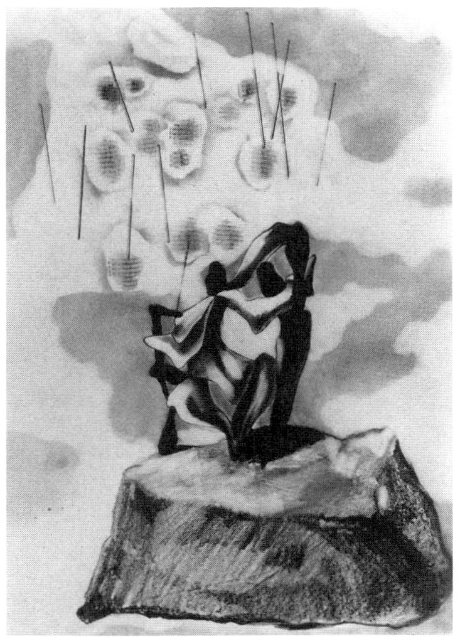

After the Flood, 1929–30, pencil on paper

. . . I am awakened around daybreak (apparently in a dream) by someone banging on the gate (I'm in Čermná) — a Gypsy woman holding a child in her arms enters my room and begins to blackmail me for some infraction — she claims I have a rifle even though my firearms permit has expired — she threatens to report me to the police — I get angry — Toyen and several friends appear in the room — I make the morning coffee for them and cook *meat* for the Gypsy woman to win her over — — — — later I go with her to the forest — I tell Toyen that I'll be back in half an hour — When we reach Jansov's "shack" I'm extremely nervous because the half-hour is up. At a bend in the path a giant Toyen appears — she is at least 10 meters high and is calling me — the Gypsy woman takes fright and hops up a rock like a SQUIRREL and disappears — the rock is damp — — — Again I am in the house with the Gypsy woman — I go out with her onto the front porch — the child runs around the porch — I shout at him not to fall into the water — the house is surrounded by water as if it were Noah's Ark — — — I'm with the Gypsy woman at some ruins and I ask her to model for me — only now do I really see her — she is about 40 years old — she agrees and asks for payment in advance — When I give it to her she goes off somewhere and returns with a spade, *digs up a patch of earth, turns it over*, then sits down on it, adopting a quaint pose, and begins to breastfeed her child, who looks to be about 8 years old — — —

X

Dream of Mother Earth

This dream is related to "Dream of the Gypsy Woman"

(1940)

I was reading Mácha's *May* before falling asleep. I was extremely tired — dozing off —

— — — beautiful earth, beloved earth,
my cradle, my grave, my mother.

Appearing to me was the very same *furrowed earth* from "Dream of the Gypsy Woman."

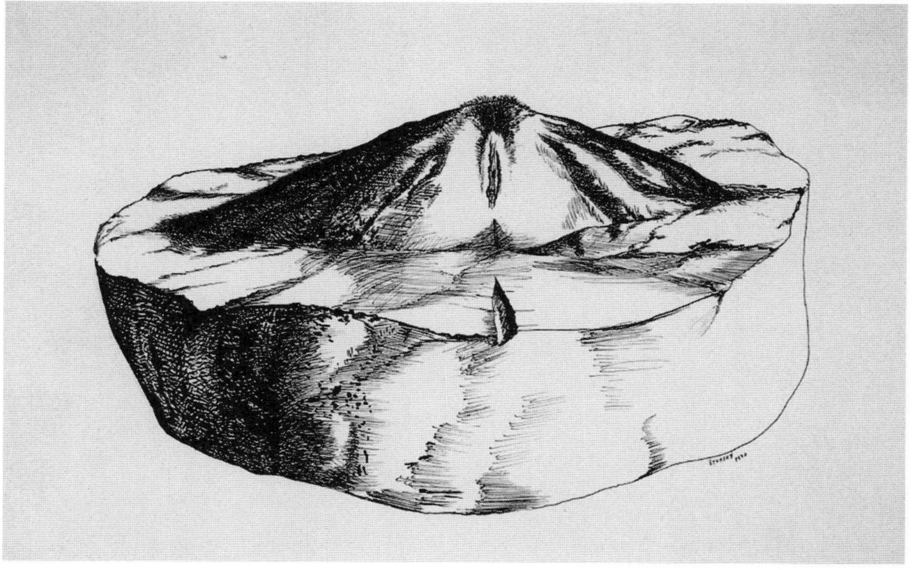

Dream of Mother Earth I, 1940, pen and ink on paper

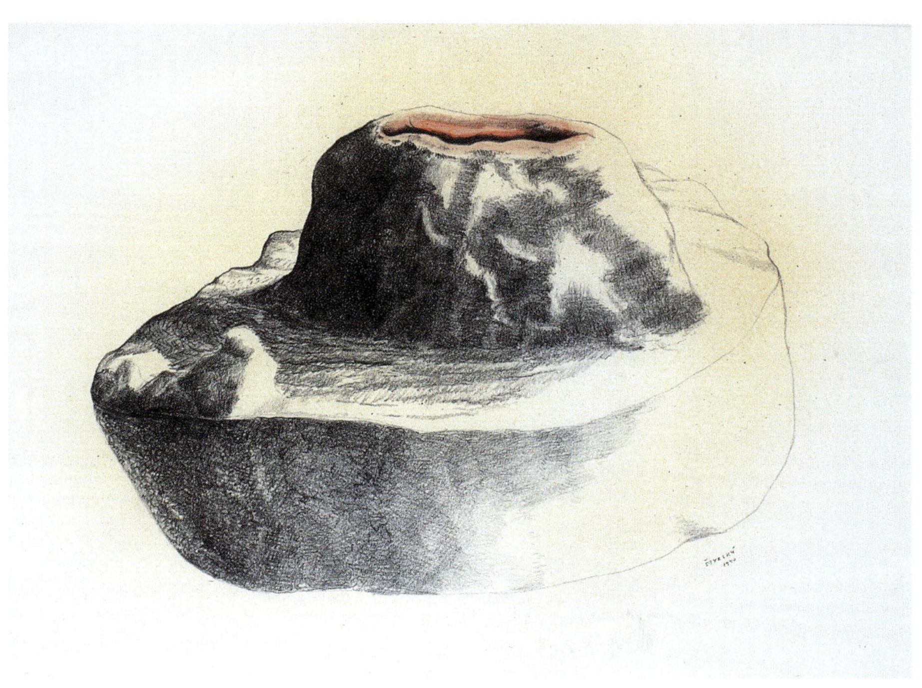

Dream of Mother Earth II, 1940, pencil and pastel on paper

XI

Dream of the Tattooed Infant

(JUNE 3, 1929)

I am with Jindřich Honzl at a dance at the Budiš Inn in Verměřovice. We're enjoying ourselves. There is a plot against us. We intend to secretly slip away. At night we flee through the garden, through fields of beet and potato. We hide in a thicket in the woods.

Honzl and I are bound to poles or to beams in the middle of a barn or a gym. Around us in an orgy of dance are ten- to twelve-year-old TATTOOED BOYS. They are armed with sticks and make threatening gestures at us. In their midst we also see an infant TATTOOED WITH PORNOGRAPHIC images.

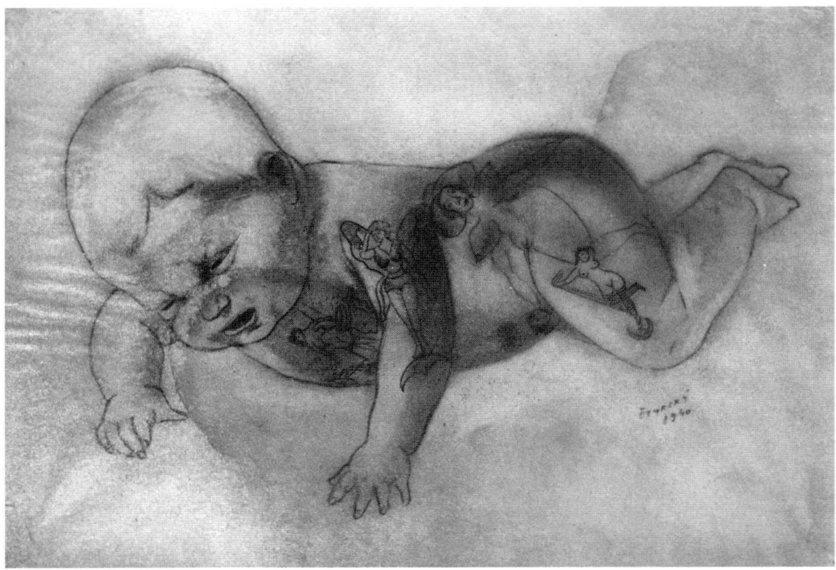

Dream Record, reconstructed, 1940, pencil and pastel on paper

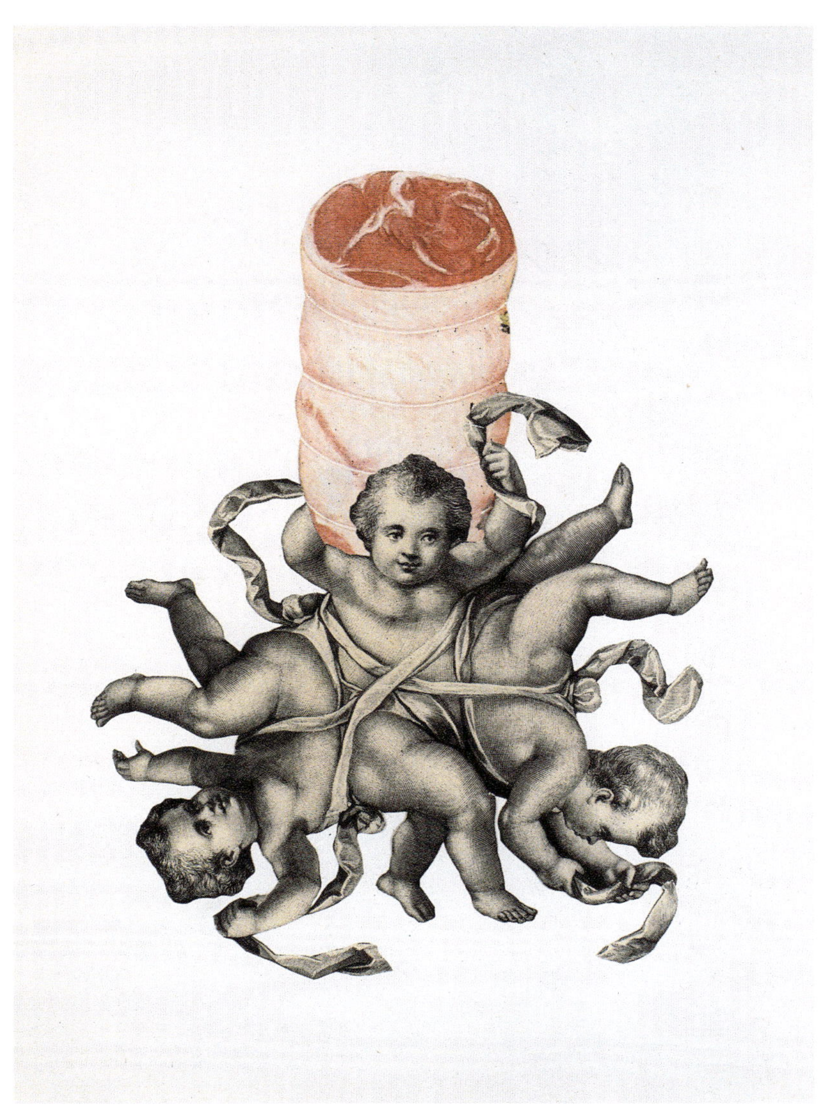

Cluster of Grapes, 1934, collage on paper

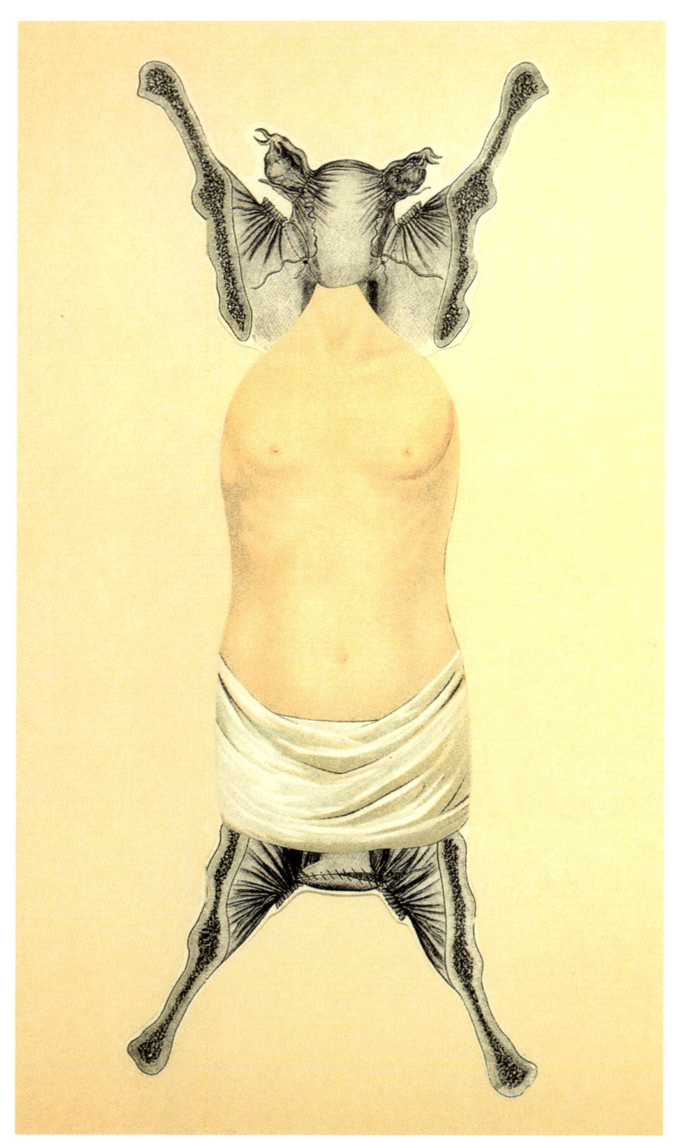

A Beautiful Baby, 1934, collage on paper

XII

Dream of the Mandrake

(1929)

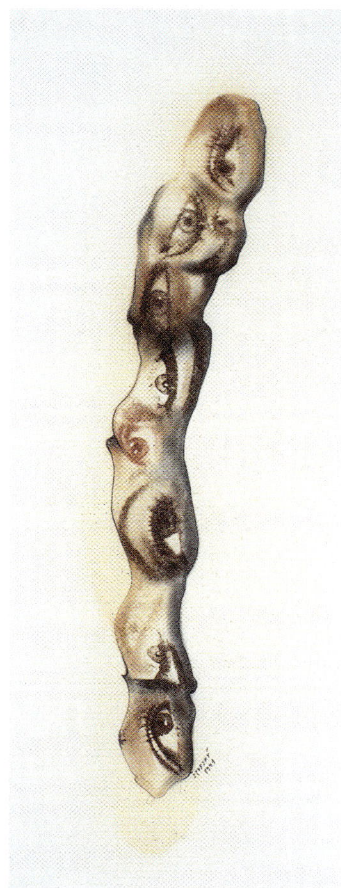

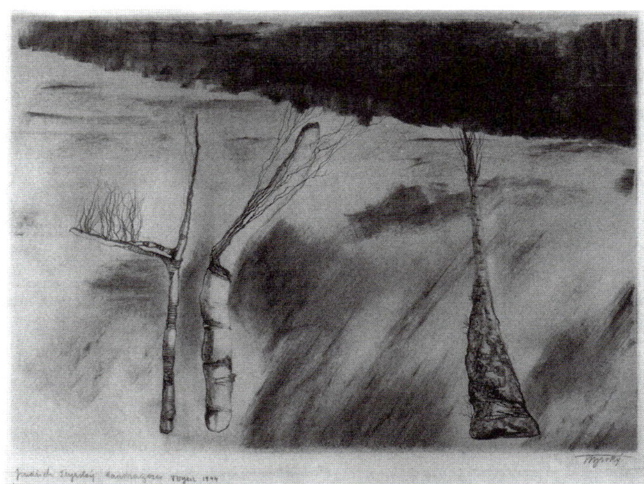

Mandrake, 1929, pencil on paper

The Omnipresent Eye XVIII (Dream of the Mandrake), 1941, ruddle on paper

XIII

Dream of Father

(THE NIGHT OF OCTOBER 15–16, 1931, KŘEMENCOVÁ ST., PRAGUE)

. . . I am at the farm in Čermná in what we call the front room. I am looking for a legal document or letter in an old writing desk. I am alone in the house, and the feeling of total isolation makes me uncomfortable. I am afraid, a type of fear I used to have as a child when I had to go alone to the cellar or attic. Suddenly the door opens and Father comes in. At this moment I feel much better. Breathing a sigh, the sensation of suffocating leaves me. In futility we both look for receipts from the sale of hay. We argue, and our arguing turns into a brawl. I see my father grow pale, his left arm raise up and hold a chair over my head, ready to club me with it. I swerve out the way and the chair misses, its momentum carrying it to the floor. I tell myself I should leave to bring this farce to an end. I think : Father is already an old man. I go to the door but glance back. I see Father standing on one leg on the backrest of the chair, his other leg balancing in the air. He's stiff and pale, practically white. He's wearing a wedding frock and over it a white gown, a blazing candle on his left shoulder. He seems mute. His shoulders convulse, jerking as if he were racked with sobbing. Yet the look he gives me is as vicious as it was a moment ago, and I see in his eyes that he'd like to pummel me though he's unable to do so. Suddenly, I don't know how, a second chair appears under his groping leg. I see him straddle on two chair backs. They seem to be attached to his legs, and all at once he starts to come after me, taking strides several meters long. But he is still stiff, and it's not his blows I run away from, since I know he's incapable of hitting me, it's his *apparition*. He has caught me off guard, and before I manage to run out the door he chases me around the room a few times. It occurs to me that he's been long dead and that what's pursuing me is his corpse. This doubles my horror. I run down a long hallway, across the yard, below the stable and barn, and into the fields. But Father on his monstrous stilts is still on my heels. Under an oak the ground gives way beneath me, and I sink into a slough. I still flee toward the chapel though I am waist-deep in mud. When it reaches my chest, I think I'm done for and at any moment the mud will close over my head. I feel an intense hatred for Father, but am comforted by the thought that he must drown in the mire with me. I look back at him and cannot find him in the whole landscape. He's vanished. I discover that a large cork float similar to a millstone has appeared around my neck. I feel relieved because I realize I'm saved. I swim. Yet I'm certain Father hasn't drowned either, and I'm terrified that in my next dream he'll come after me again on those chairs.

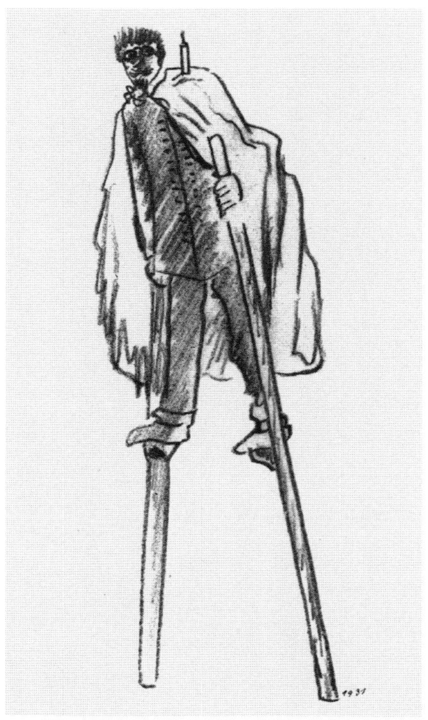

Second Dream Record, 1931, pencil on paper

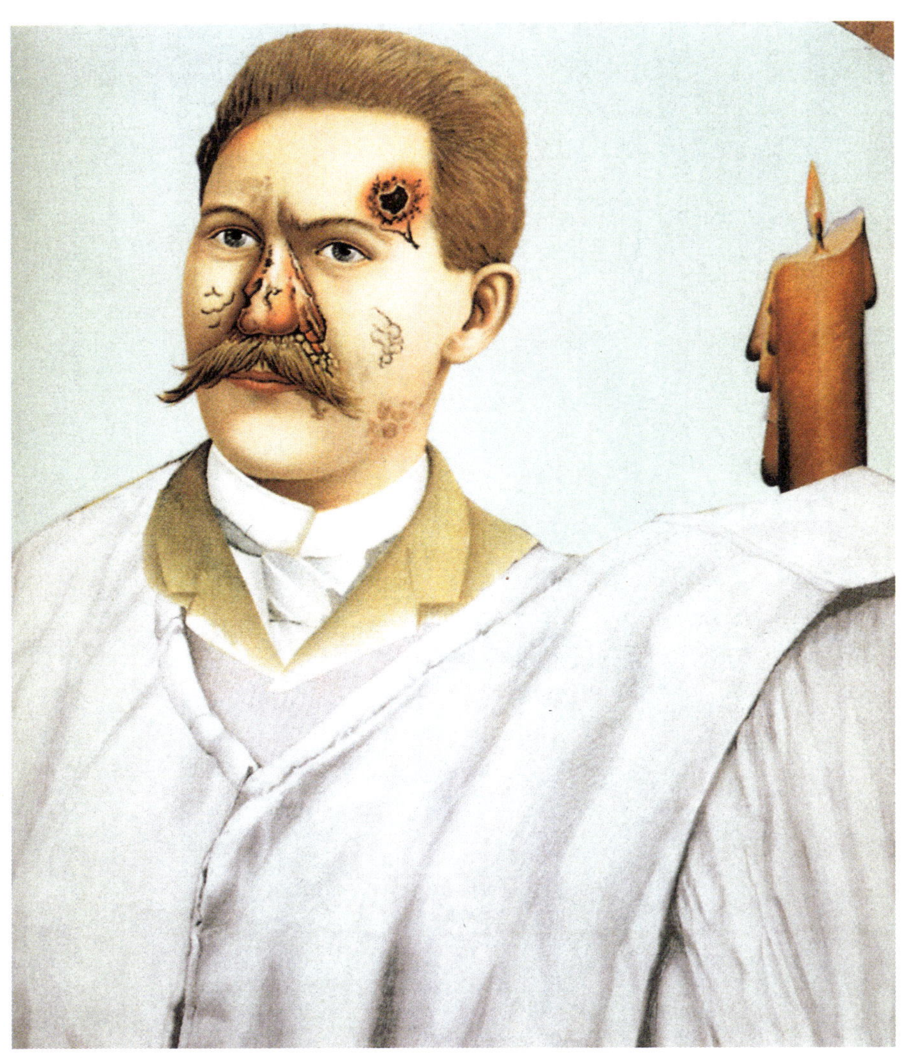

My Father, 1934, collage on paper

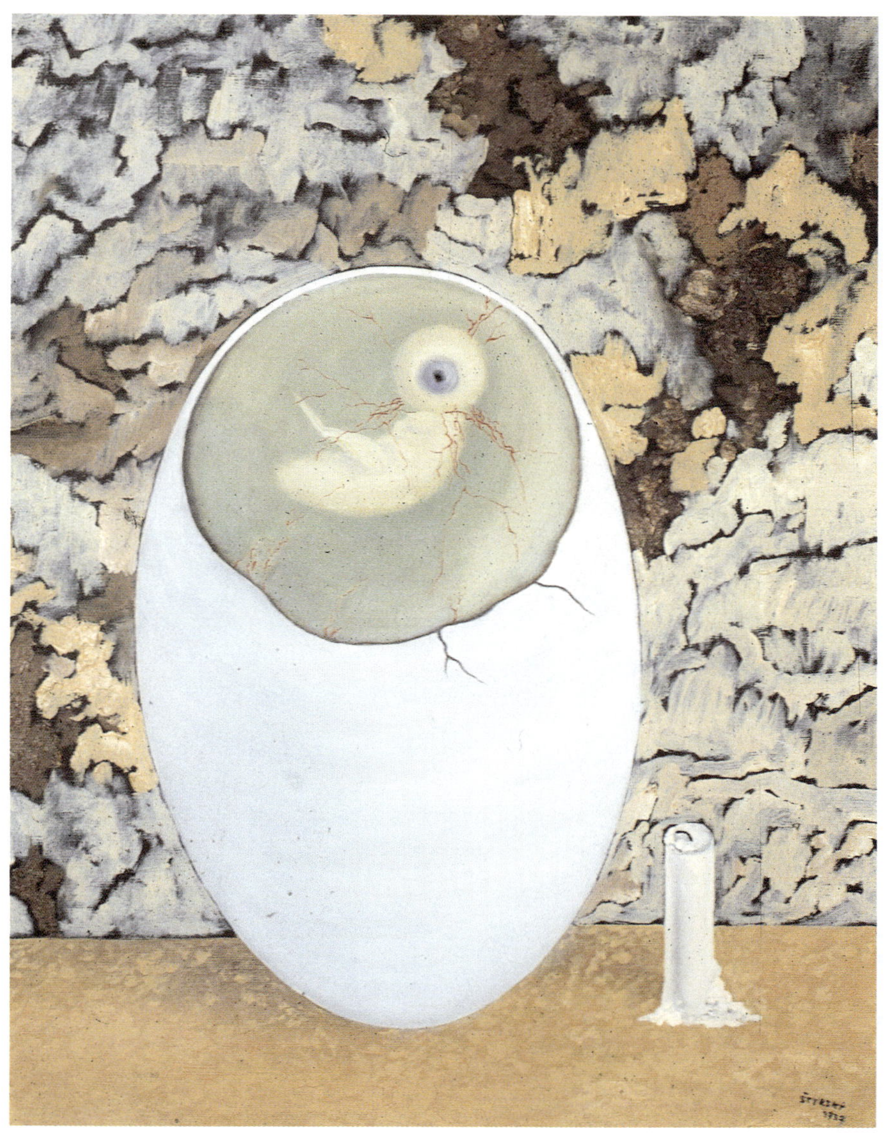

Transformation, 1937, oil on canvas

XIV

Dream of Emilie and Marta

(1931)

I am in a study at the grade school in Petrovice, tinkering with an old compass. I look out the window at the nursery of fruit trees, the bare branches of apple and pear trees covered in blossom. It's a beautiful spring day and the old women are planting potatoes in the fields behind the nursery. I am disturbed by some sort of commotion coming from the adjacent classroom (a door leads from the study to the classroom) : a woman's voice repeats over and over a medical precept, then two voices haggle over a thighbone, then quiet. I try to draw a circle in an office ledger, but the interminable silence makes me so curious I leave the study and walk into the heated, empty classroom where Marta and Karel are sitting on the last bench and kissing. Both are embarrassed and insist I stay. I feel that Marta loves me even though she's kissing Karel. I glance at the window, completely covered in snow, to the garden, where directly opposite is the iron pump, the same pump I would, as a young boy, douse with hot water whenever it froze over. And this snow-covered pump, green, in front of the snow-covered fence buries me in melancholy. Emilie in furs and someone I don't know are standing by it, waving at me. I shout : I'm coming. I open the door to the hallway — winter slaps my face — I take a seat in the sleigh and off I go with Emilie and the stranger.

XV

Dream of Butterflies

(1932 – NEARLY THE SAME DREAM IN 1937)

I was lying on a grassy balk (Čermná?). Suddenly I saw butterflies landing on the flowers around me (cabbage whites), their tiny bodies pierced by long pins as if they had flown away from a collection. Before I even realized it, an entire swarm suddenly flew to me and landed on my hands and face, until they had completely covered me, jabbing mej with their pins. I woke up in pain, and also : they would have SUFFOCATED me.

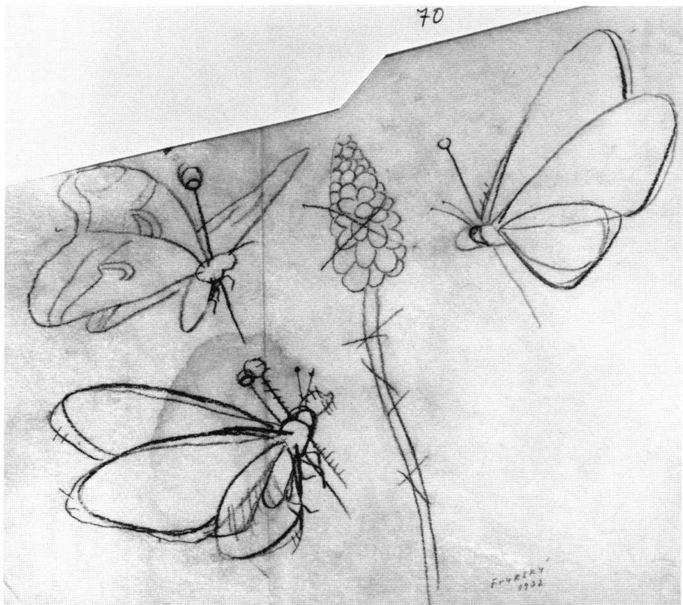

Dream Record, 1932, pencil on paper

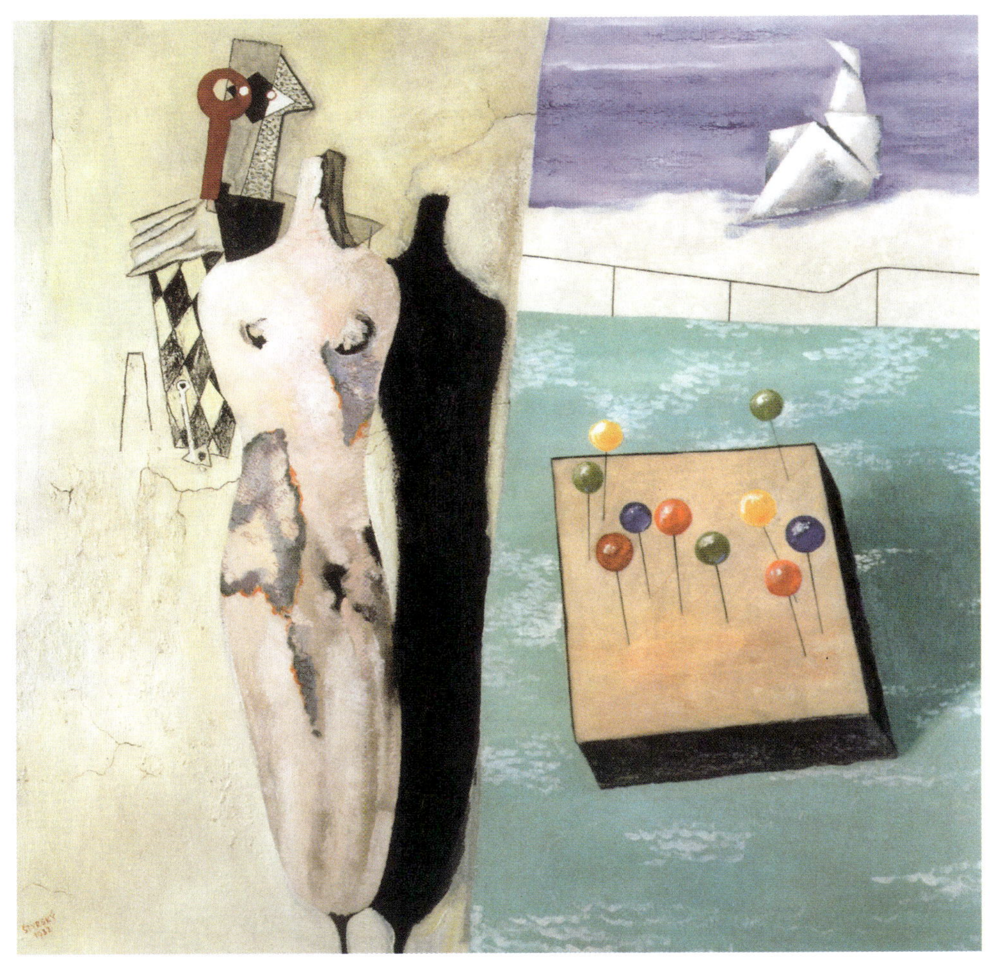

Painting, 1932, oil on canvas

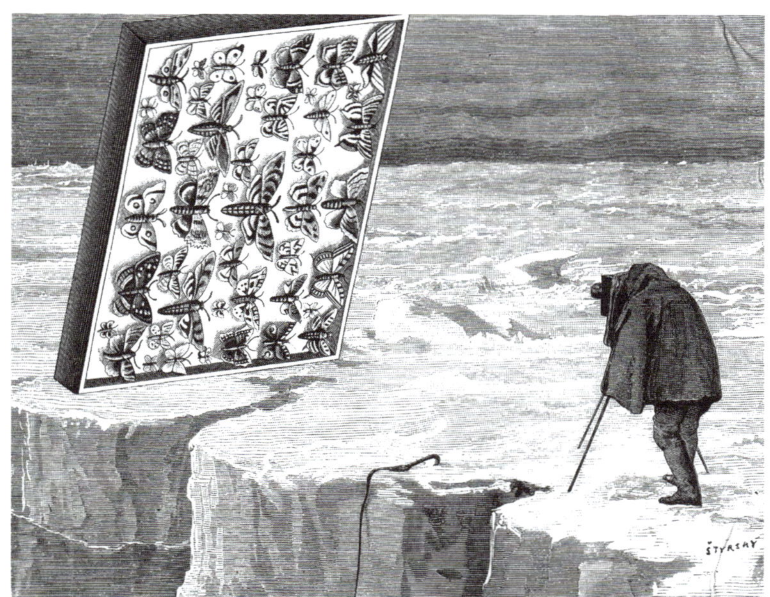

The North Pole, 1939, collage on paper

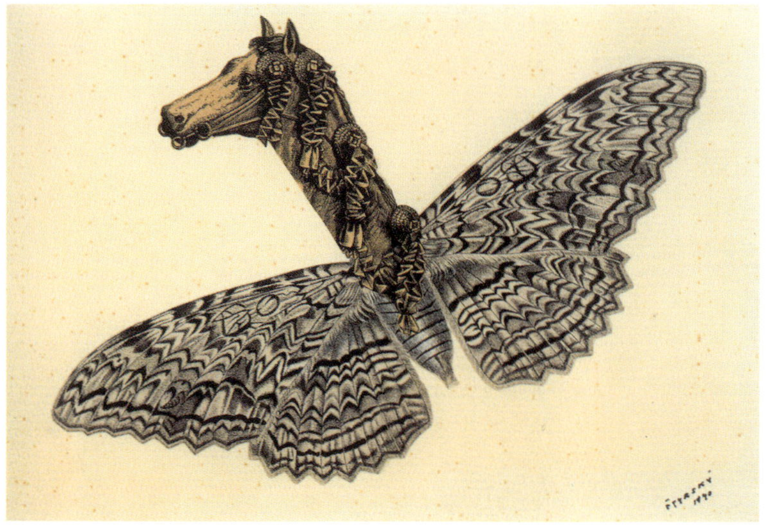

Collage, 1939, collage on paper

XVI

Dream of Scarecrows and a Birdhouse

(RECONSTRUCTION OF AN UNRECORDED DREAM FROM 1933?)

— — — I find myself in a desert (is it Harar?) with *curious rock formations* that will never be wiped from my memory. On me is a dirty gray blanket and some sort of slab with writing fastened to my back. I believe the year and manner of my death is inscribed on it. I sit on the ground hunched over, pulling the blanket around me — — — I'm sitting on a pile of whiskers that are spread out on greasy newspaper — — — — — four people in the distance are coming toward me. When I am able to make them out more clearly I notice they are not people but scarecrows, like the kind I used to see in the fields of Čermná. I run from them to the rocks, from where I will observe what they're up to. And with horror I see that one of the scarecrows is me. I see myself hoisted on a pole just like the others — — — we walk four abreast in tight formation, and stuck atop my pole (a pilgrim's staff ?) is a woman's torso, while the whole desert transforms into a volcanic field — — — — — a birdhouse is attached to the rocks — — — — then everything vanishes, and a gray bird wanders through the sand.

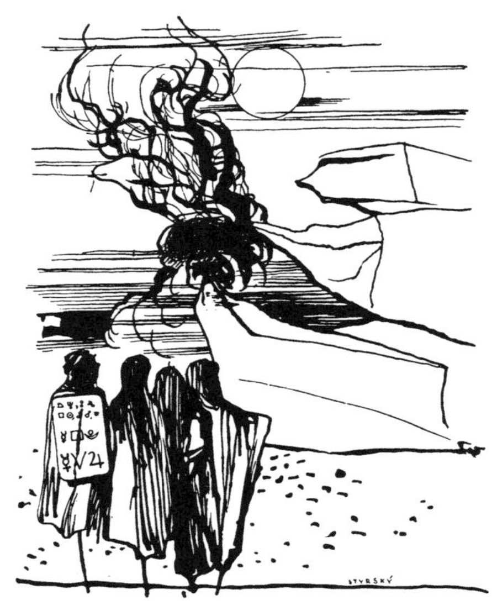

Scarecrows, 1933, pen and ink on paper

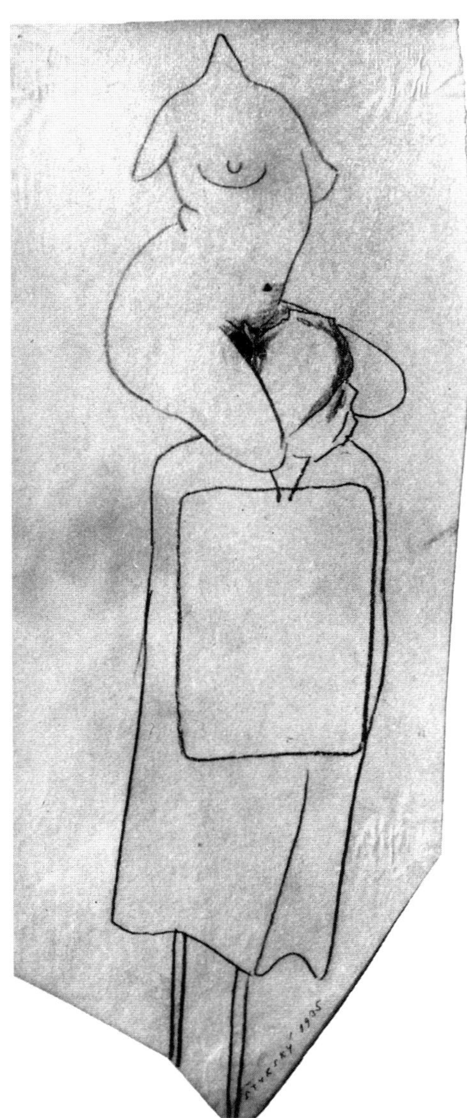

Dream of Scarecrows I, 1935, pencil on paper

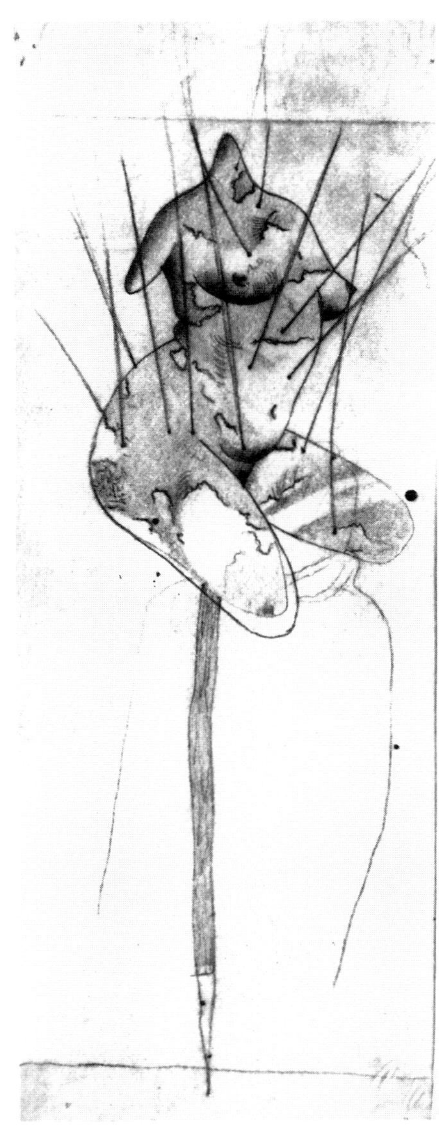

Dream of Scarecrows III, 1935, pencil on paper

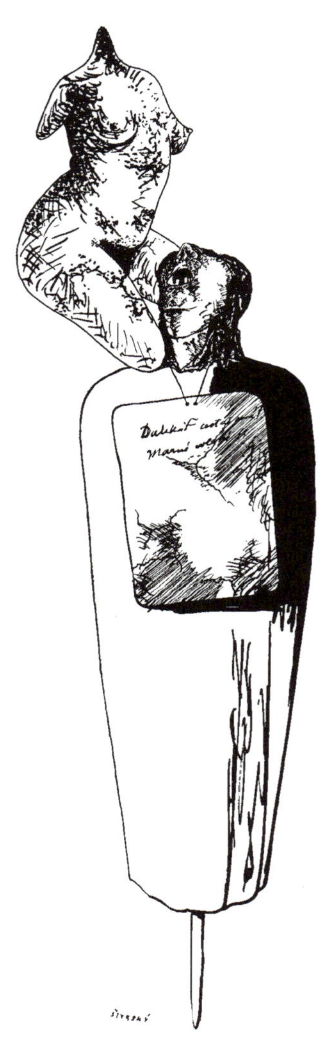

May, 1936, pen and ink on paper

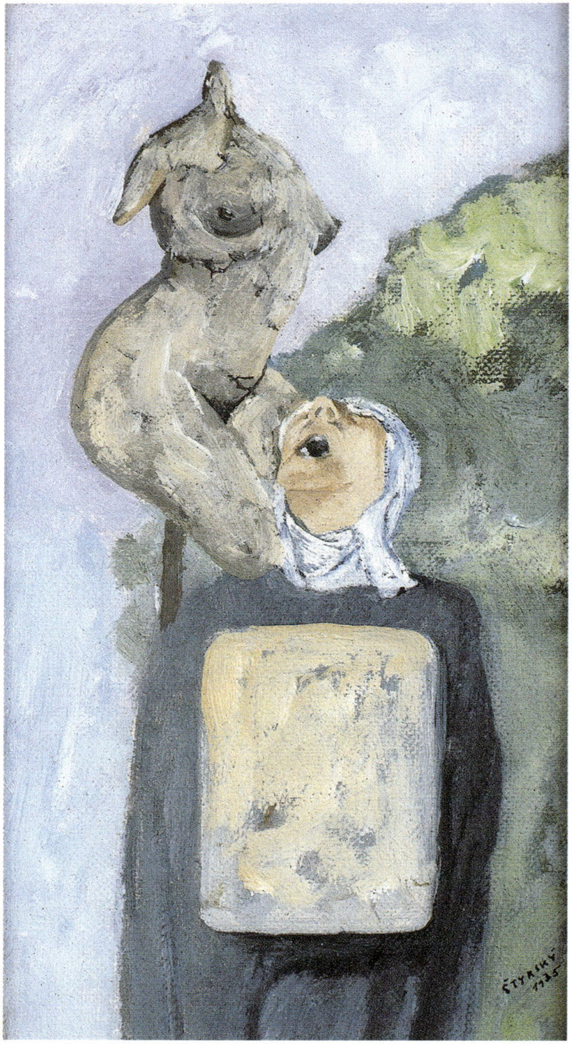

A Dream ("Long is my journey! Futile cry!!"), 1935, oil on canvas

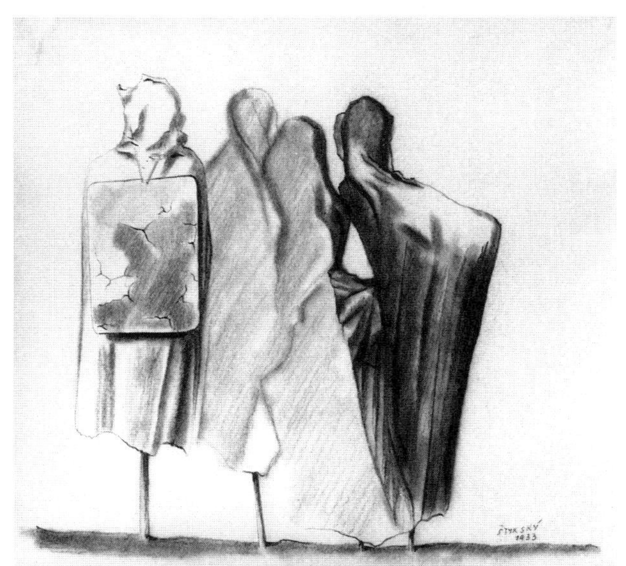

Scarecrows, 1933, pencil on paper

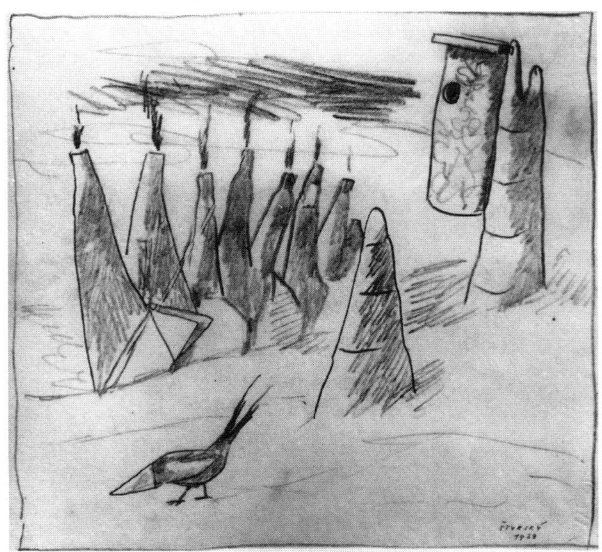

Sketch for *The Year 1939*, 1939, pencil on paper

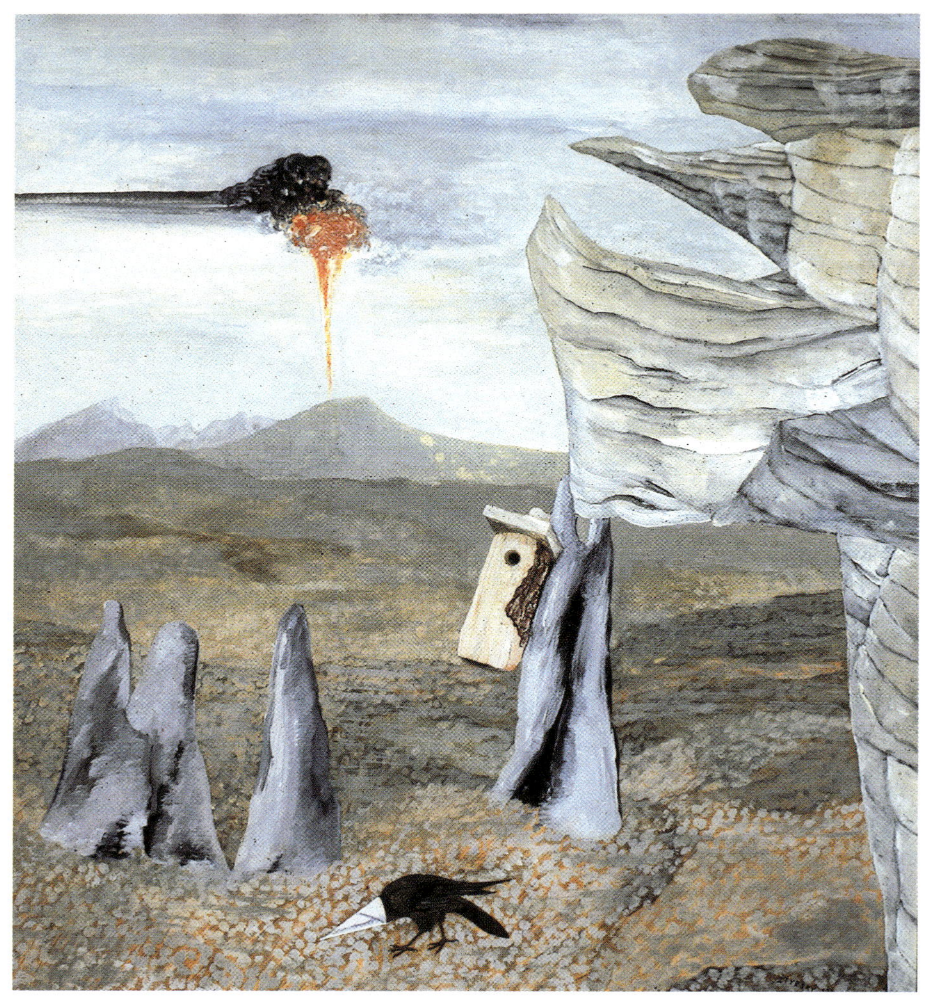

The Year 1939, 1939, oil on canvas

XVII

Dream of Jaroslav Seifert

(NIGHT OF JULY 22–23, 1934, HOTEL PROKOP, ŠPIČÁK NA ŠUMAVĚ)

Dusk. We're walking through a terrifying forest. Through a tunnel we come to a quarry. No way out. It is night, but moonlit. A child whose age and sex I cannot determine is running and jumping along the rocks. I'm extremely worried the child will not be able to walk further. He howls that he's thirsty. He's Jaroslav Seifert's son. Ura brings water in one of those square glasses countryfolk use for drinking wine. Seifert is furious. He says children should always have fruit juice mixed with their water. He catches his kid and holds him between his knees in the same way one holds a goose when feeding it. With one swipe he lops off the head. Then he comes to us. He's squeezing the child's head in his hands. I find the whole scene comical. Seifert's gestures remind me of a salon magician. He shows us a wrinkled lemon. Ura holds out the glass and tells him to give the lemon a good squeeze. I regret that it's night and I cannot photograph Seifert for my album of Czech poets.

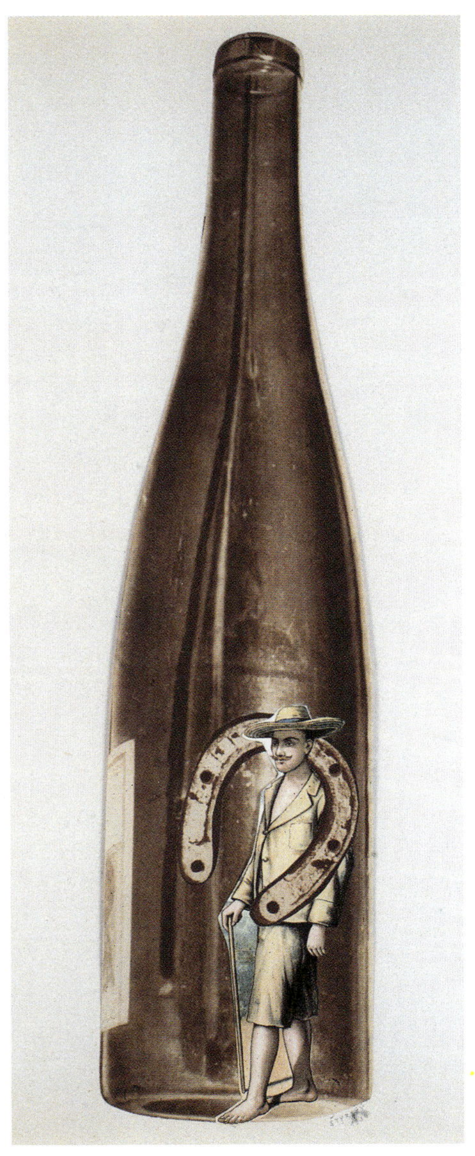

Dream of Jaroslav Seifert, 1934, collage on paper

XVIII

Dream of Breasts

(1934 – OCTOBER 28)

— listen to the milk PURLING inside her as she walks — — — — —

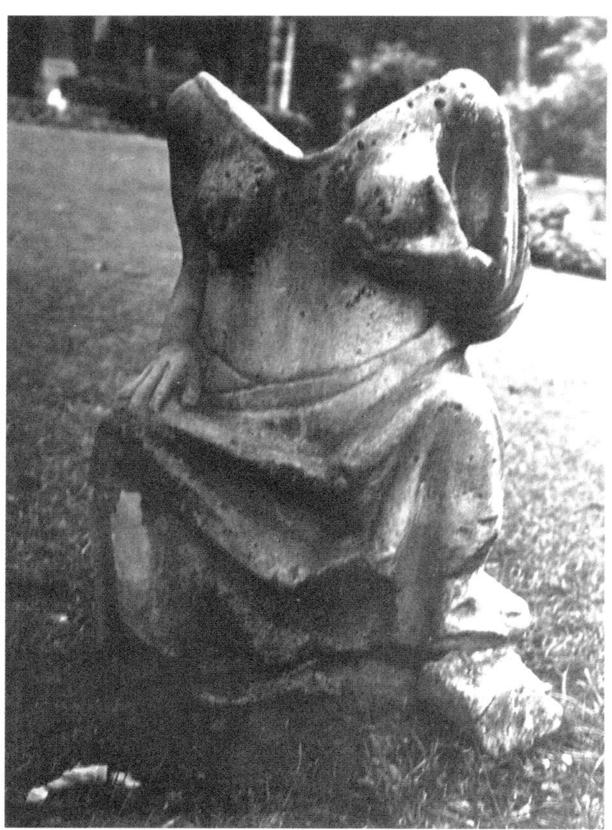

Photograph from the garden of the Musée de Cluny in Paris

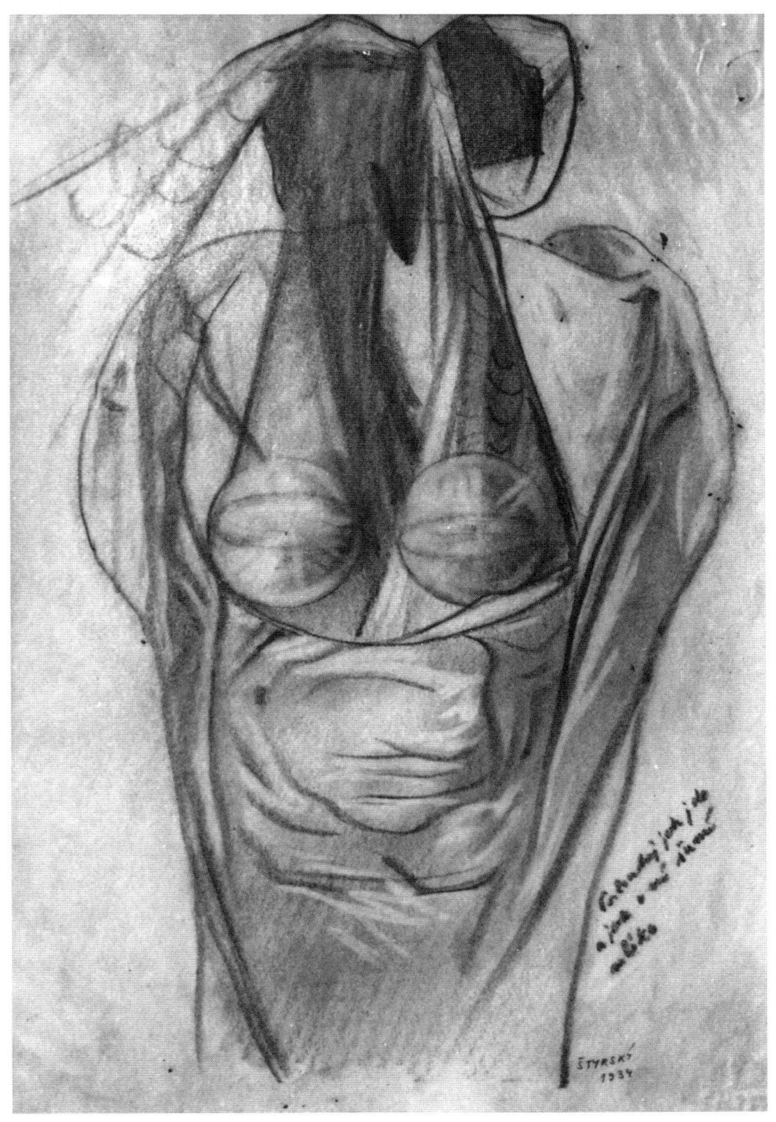

Sketch for *Person Withering at the Hip*, 1934, pencil on paper

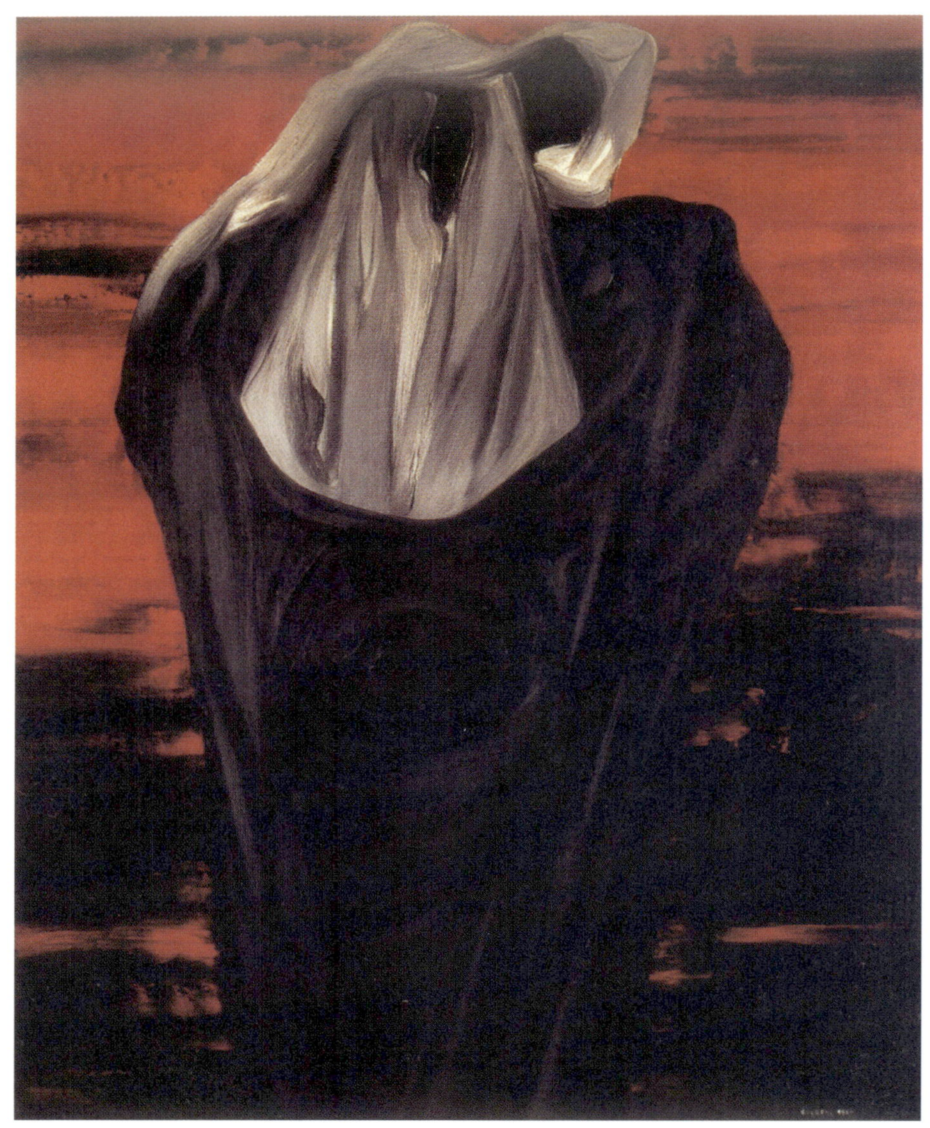

Person Withering at the Hip, 1934, oil on canvas

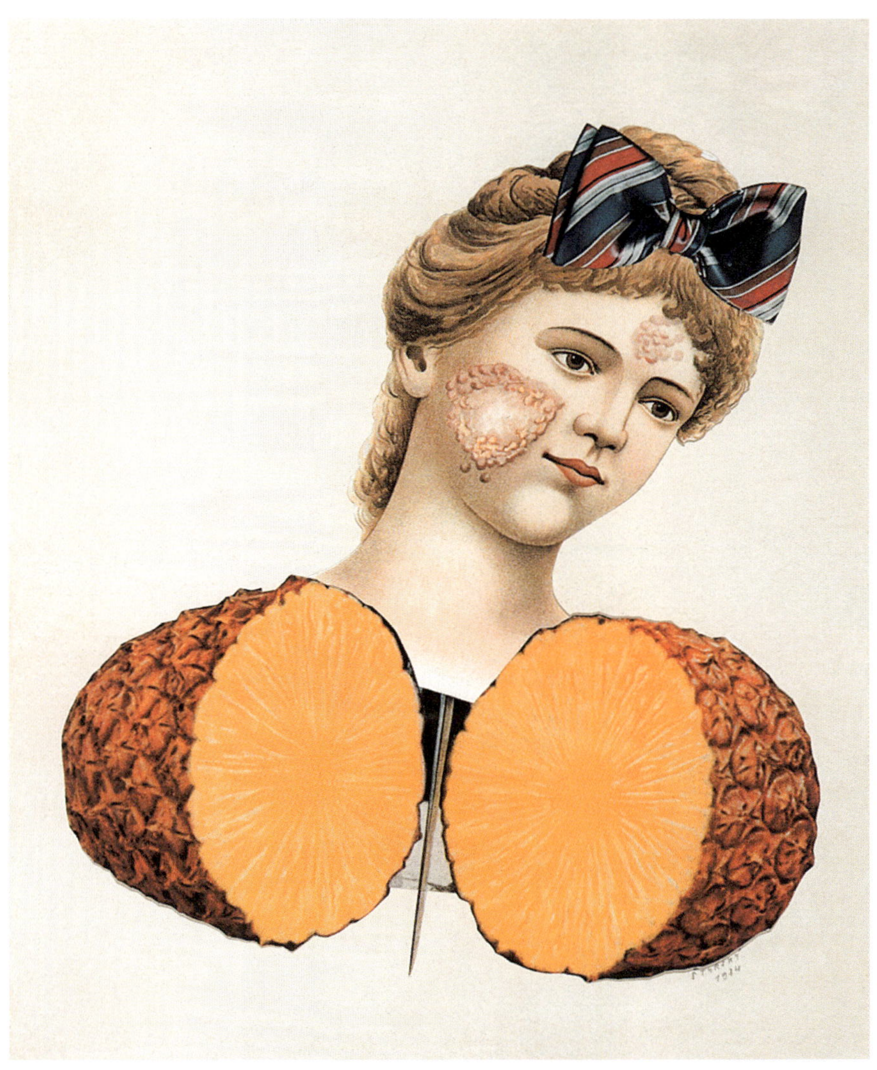

Coffee Doll I, 1934, collage on paper

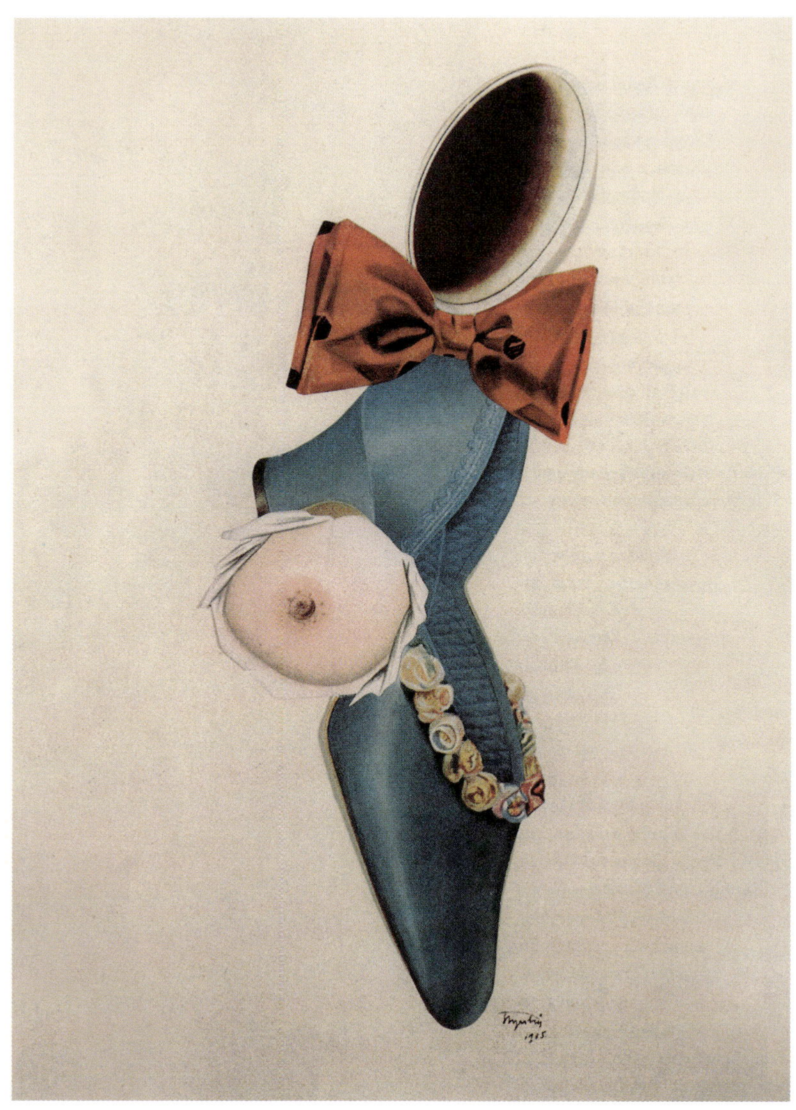

Coffee Doll II, 1935, collage on paper

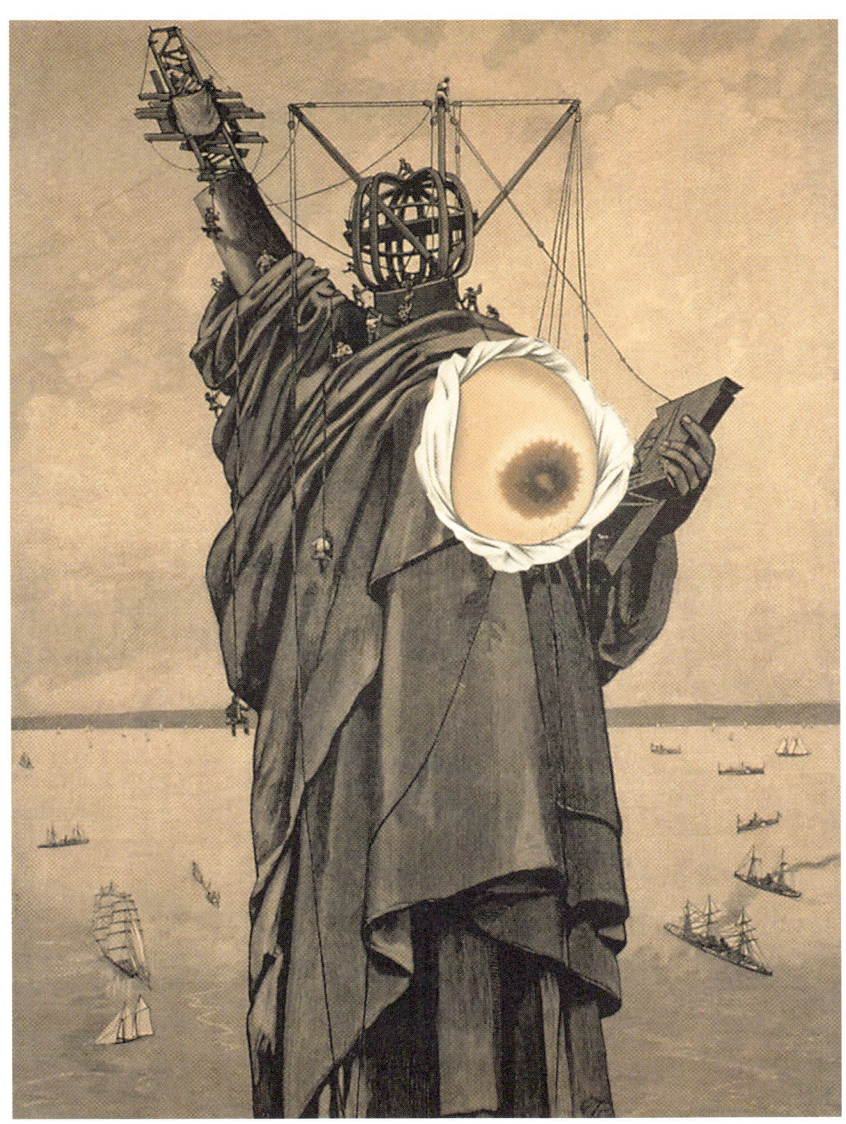

The Statue of Liberty, 1934, collage on paper

XIX

A Dream

(1934)

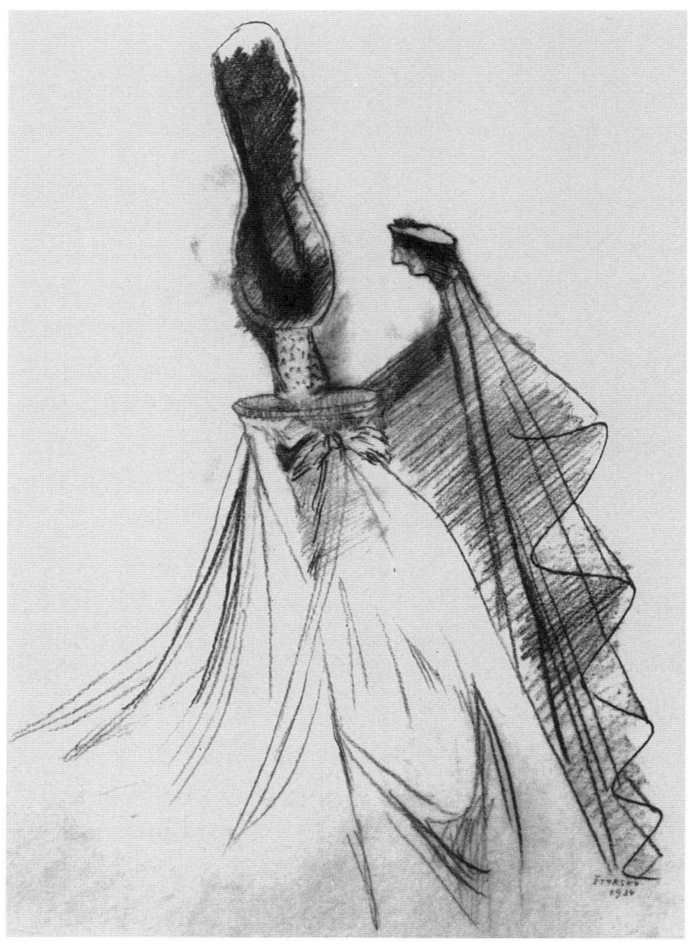

Dream Record, 1934, pencil on paper

XX

Scatological Dreams

(1934)

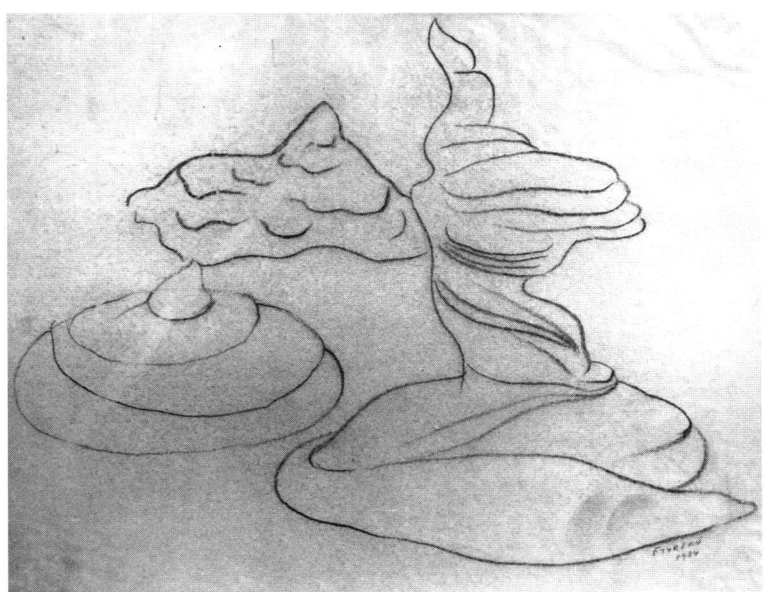

Scatological Dream Record I, 1934, pencil on paper

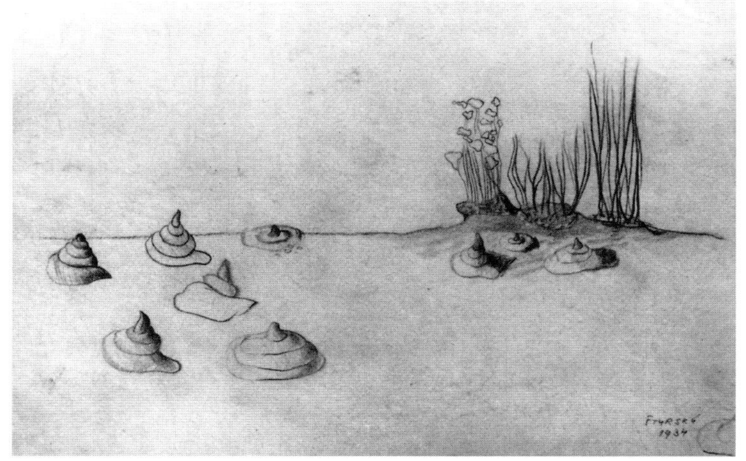

Scatological Dream Record II, 1934, pencil on paper

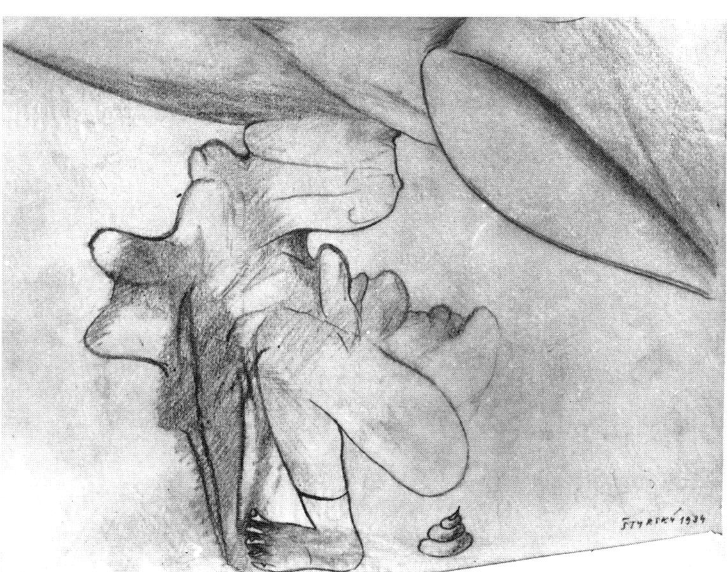

Scatological Dream Record III, 1934, pencil on paper

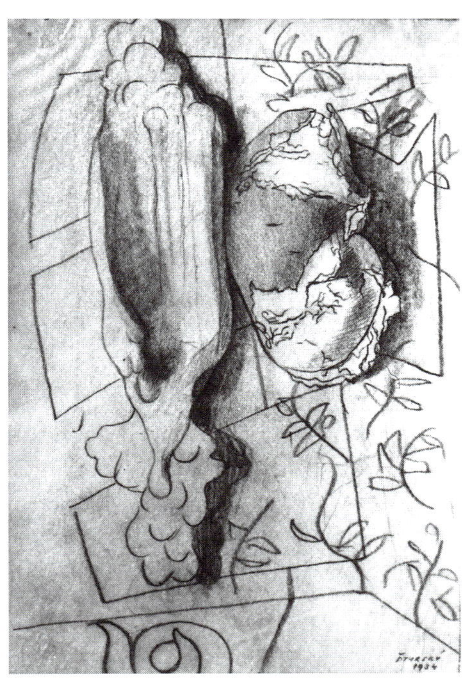

Study for *Runny Doll*, 1934, pencil on paper

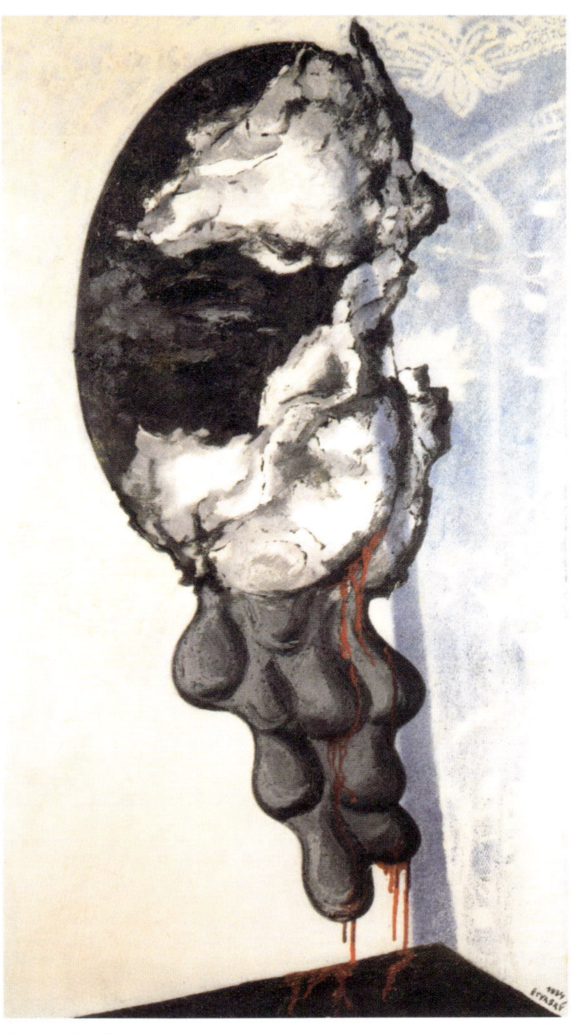

Runny Doll, 1934, oil on canvas

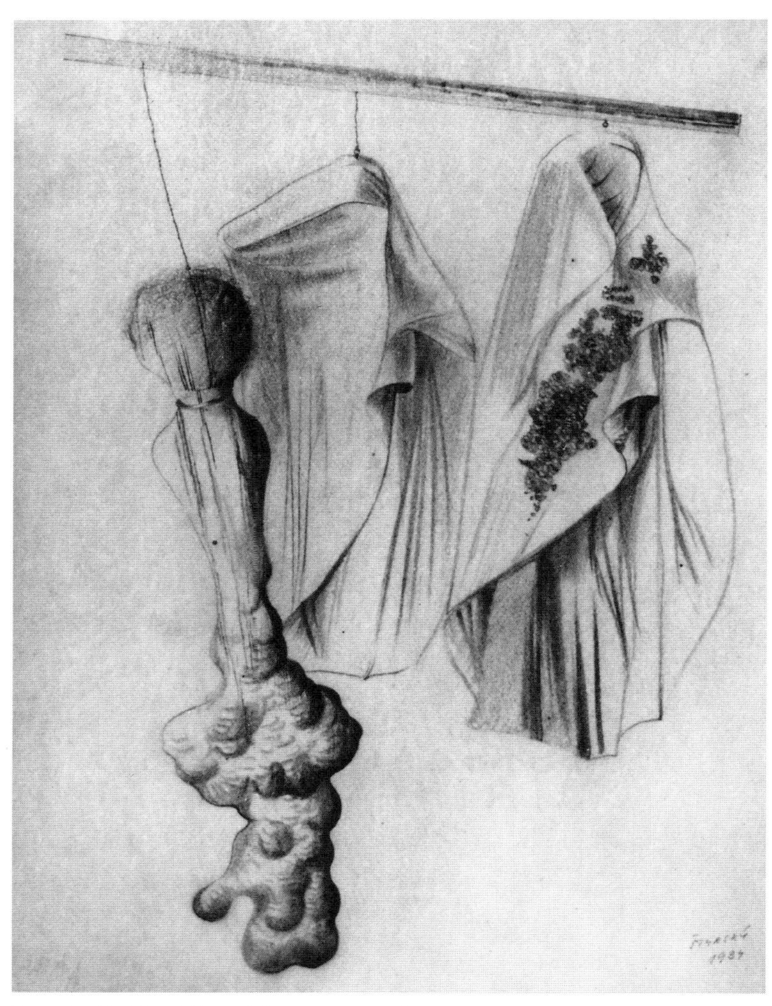

Drawing for *Windblown Man*, 1934, pencil on paper

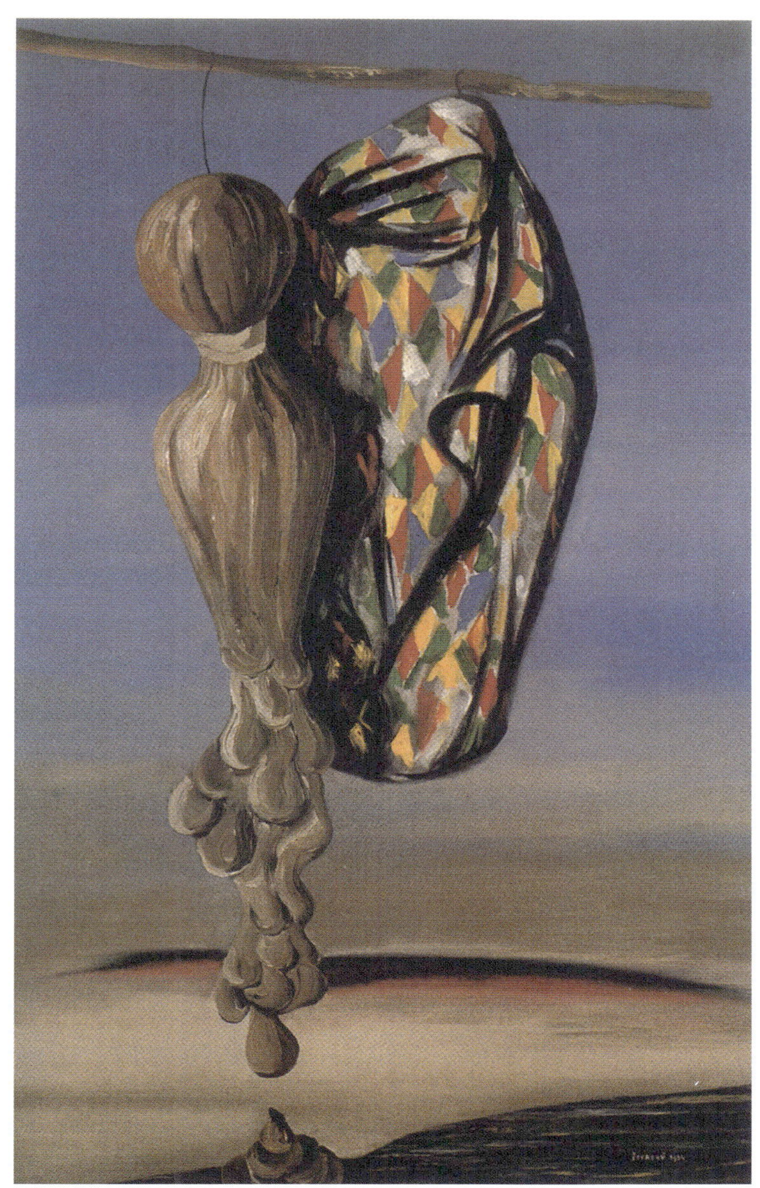

Windblown Man, 1934, oil on canvas

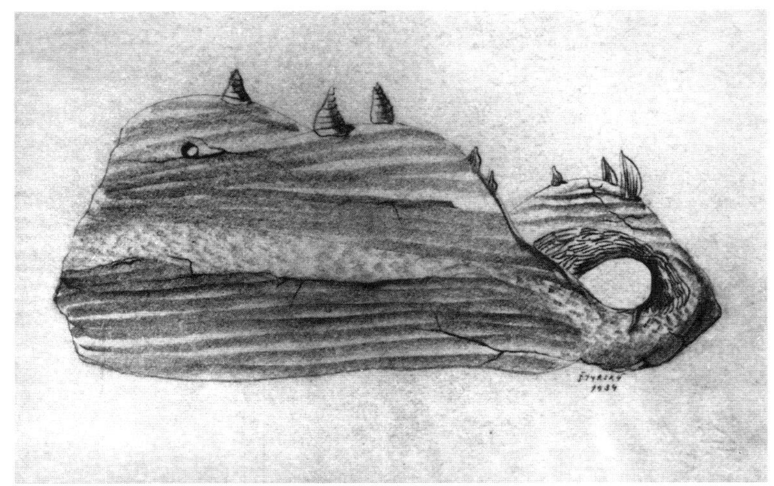

Sketch for *Sodom and Gomorrah*, 1934, pencil on paper

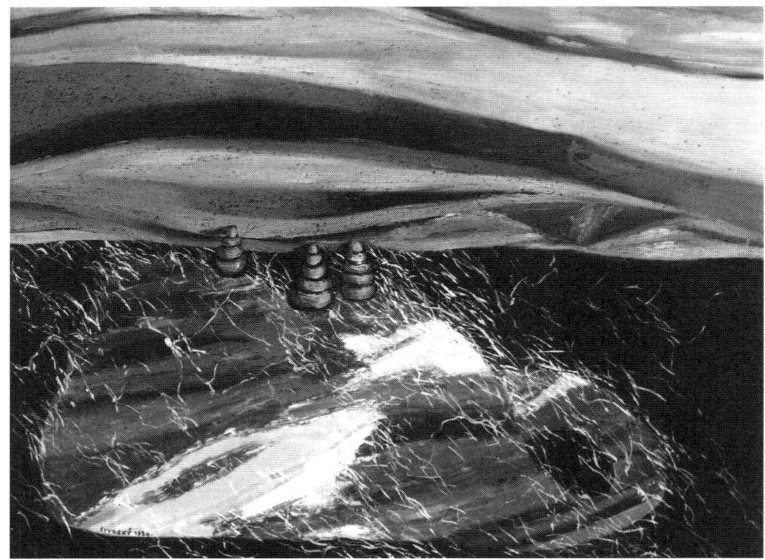

Sodom and Gomorrah, 1934, oil on canvas

XXI

Dream of the Bearded Head

(1936)

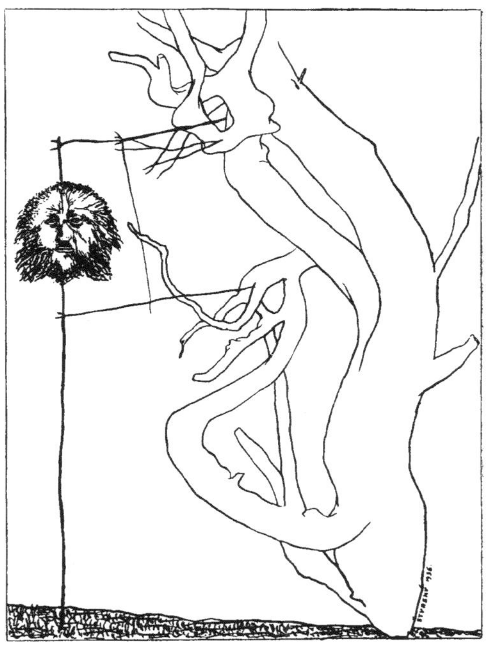

Study I, 1936, pen and ink on paper

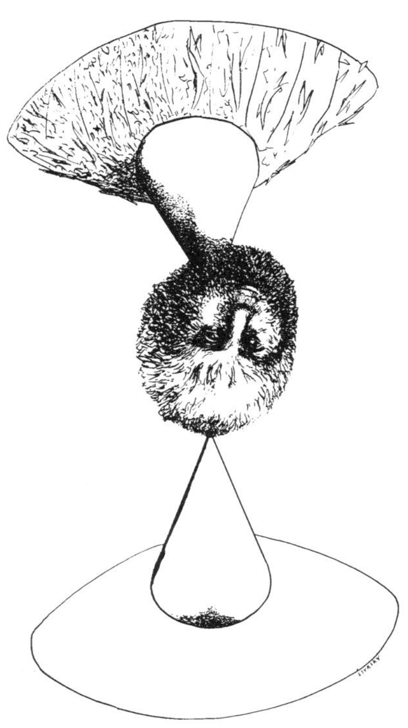

Spain, 1936, pen and ink on paper

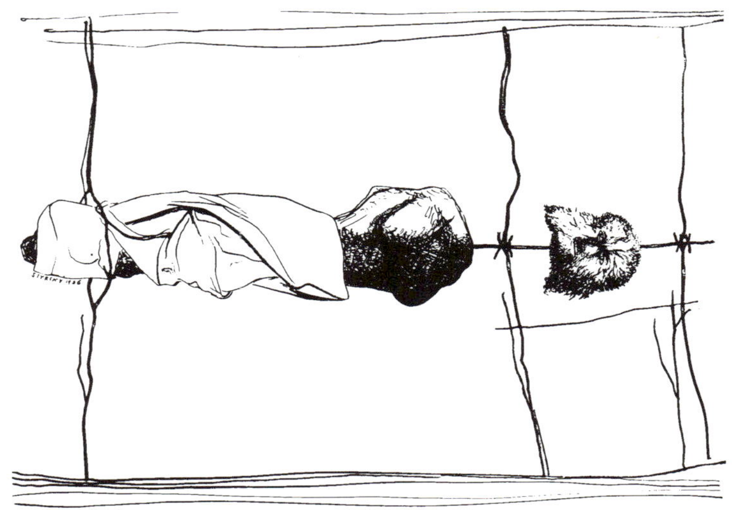

Study II, 1936, pen and ink on paper

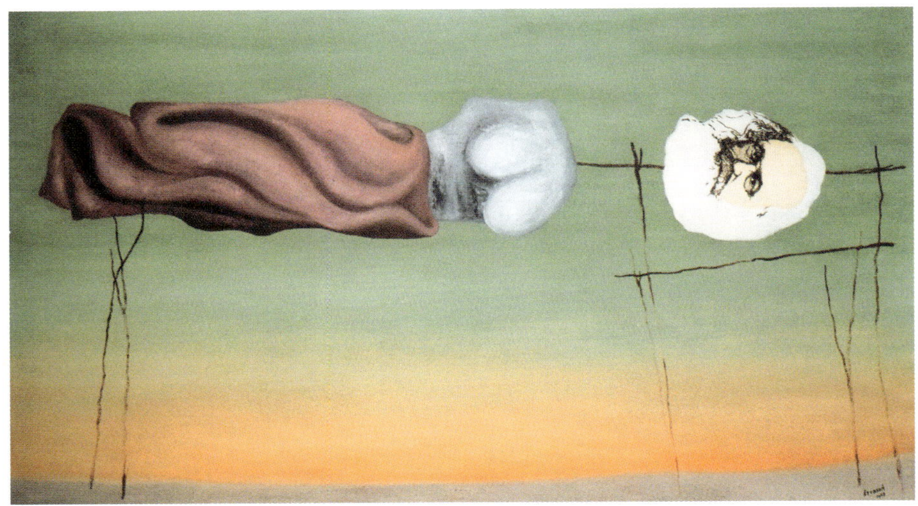

Homage to Karl Marx, 1937, oil on canvas

XXII

Dream of the Vest and the Grafted Tree

(1937)

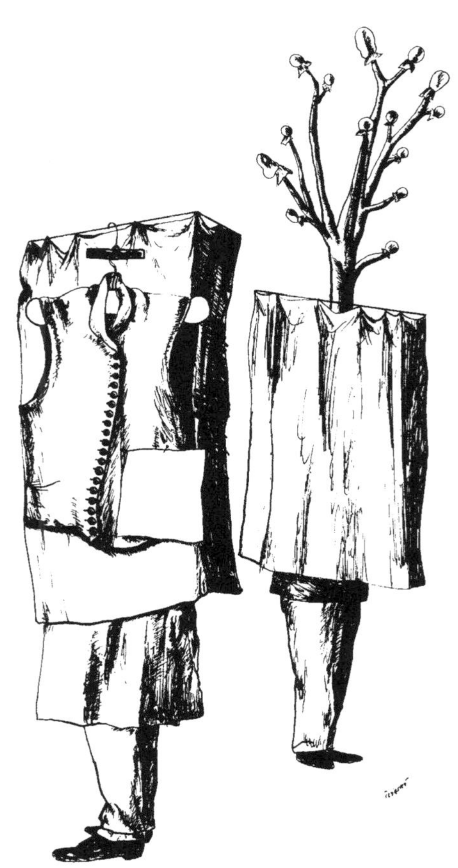

Dream Record, 1937, pen and ink on paper

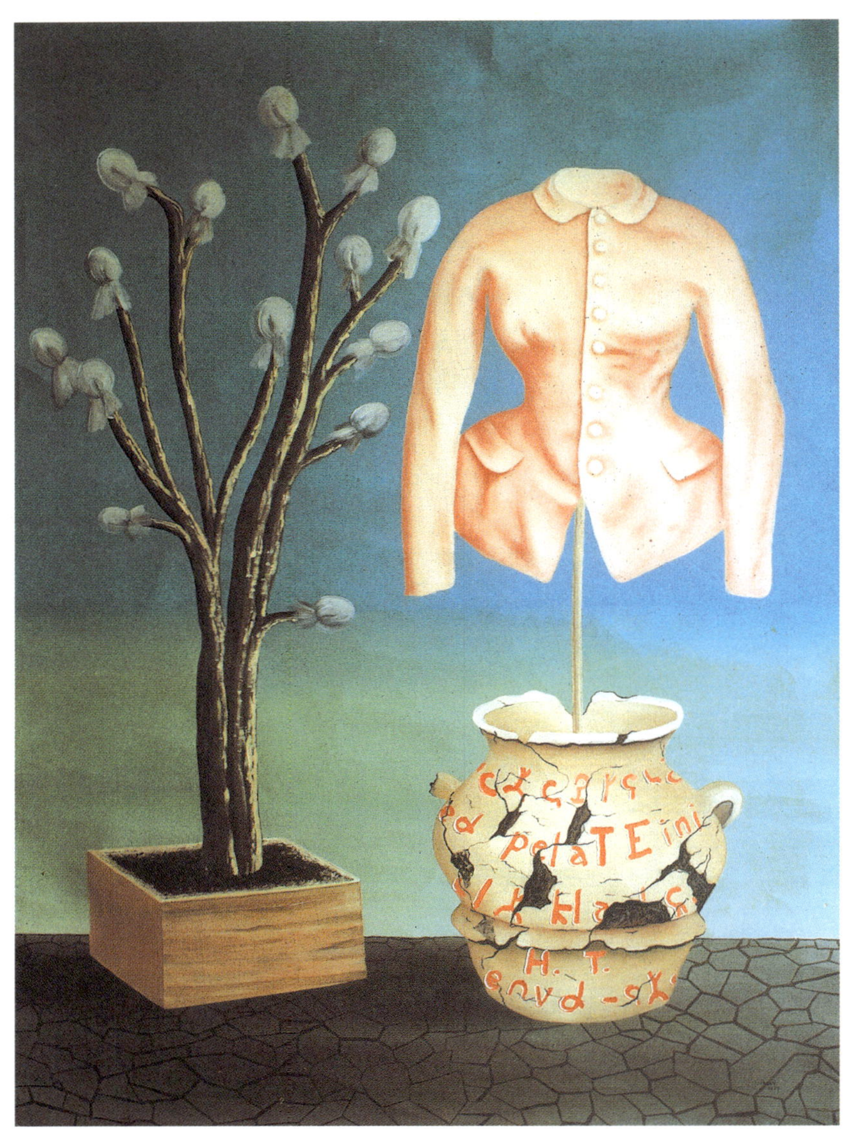

Melancholy, 1937, oil on canvas

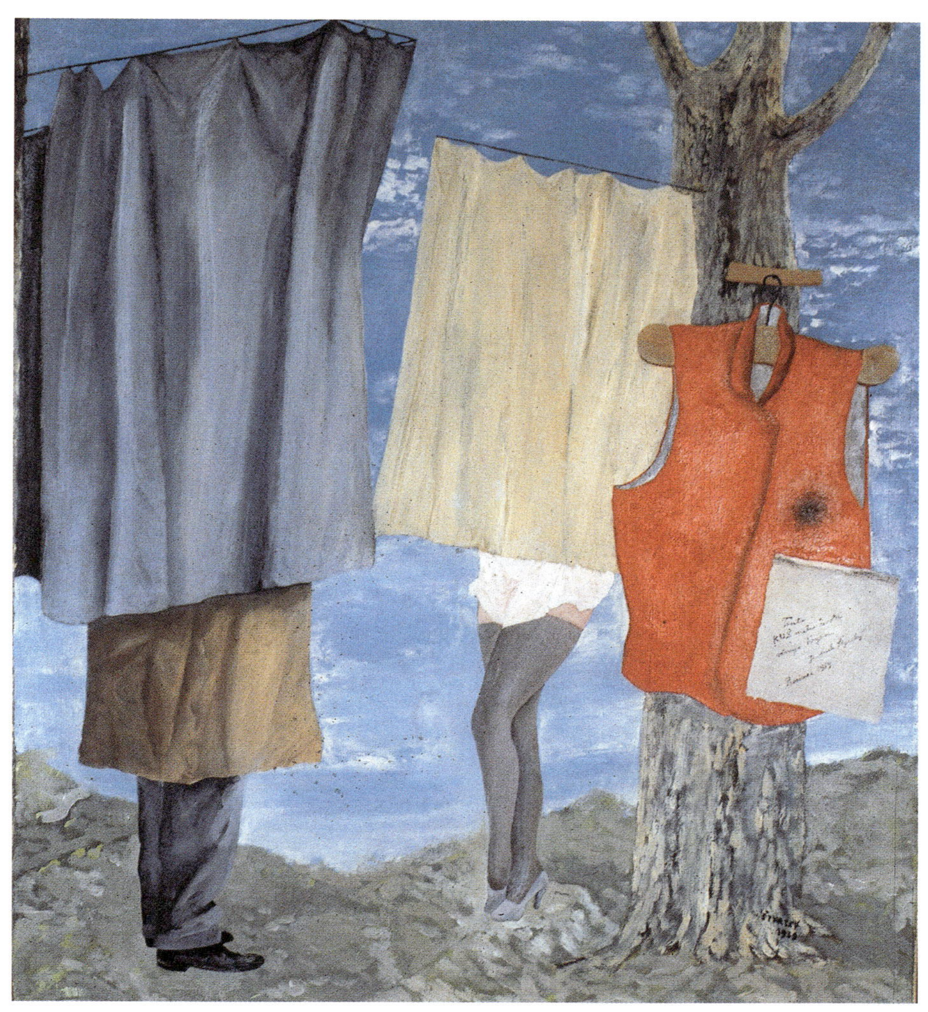

Mayakovsky's Vest, 1939, oil on canvas

XXIII

Dream of Books

(1937)

We are in Paris and getting ready to leave for Prague. Before we go I would like to browse the bouquinistes. Toyen tells me to find her a book to pass the time with on the train. When I come to the embankment I realize that the bookstalls are no longer in their usual places and have been set up instead along the edges of the city's bridges.

The bridges also aren't in their usual places, and there are more of them. Eventually I find several familiar booksellers. One of them has a number of books on the ground. "New purchases," he tells me. I rummage through the books until I find three of peculiar size : long and thin.* They are from the 18th century and filled with exquisite engravings, colored, depicting tropical plants, palms, and trees. I buy them and quickly walk away before the bouquiniste reconsiders. To my mind, I've cheated him. I'm also mindful not to miss my train. Toyen is at the station by now. But I cannot help going to Notre-Dame to see a well-known bookseller from whom I've made some stellar purchases in the past. I stop by his stall and pull out an old leather-bound volume at random. When I look at it, I see a crumpled ear on the front cover, and when I take the book from its row, the ear straightens out. I steal a glance at the bookseller sitting behind me. In front of him is a stool with a laver of water. He removes one *eared* book after another from the shelves, dusting off the ears and then giving them a good washing, after which he dries them with a clean towel. — — — — The ears flower — — —

* Around 15 x 35 cm, author's note, 1941.

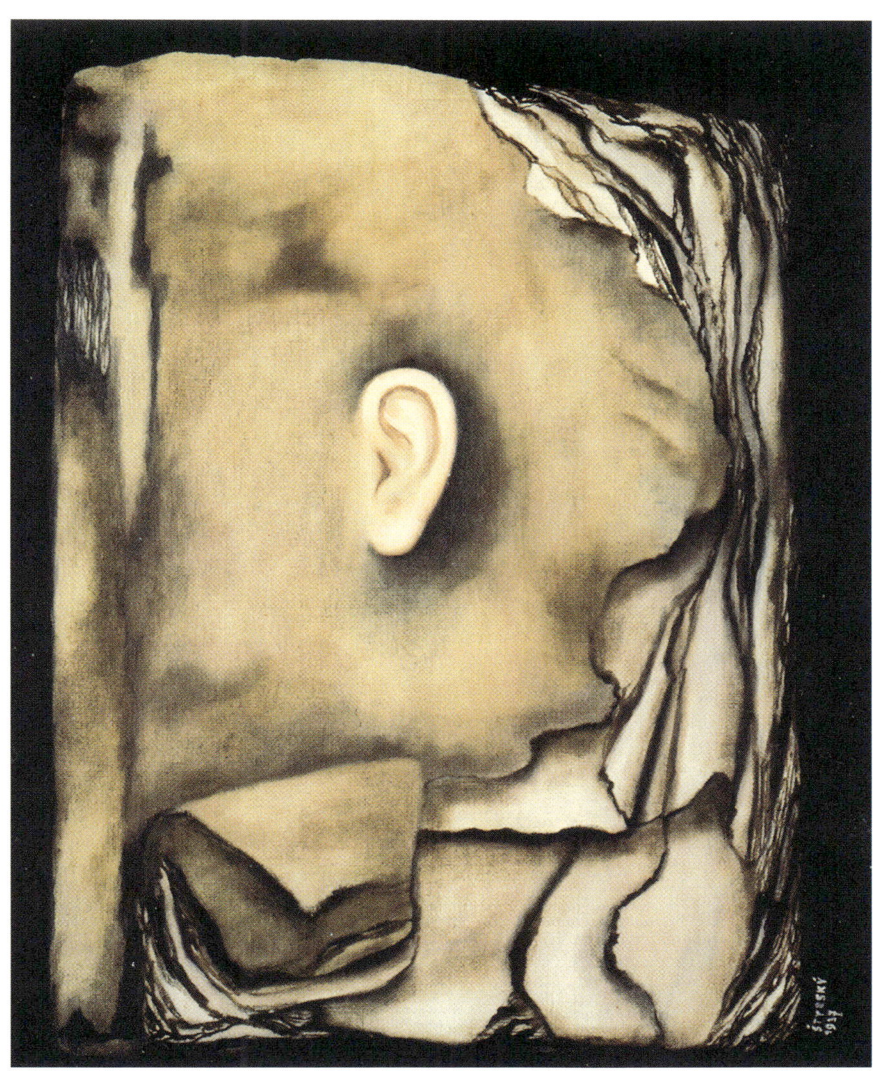

The Gift, 1937, oil on canvas

XXIV

Dream of the Sack

(1937)

— — — When I wanted to untie the sack to see what was inside, I woke up — — —

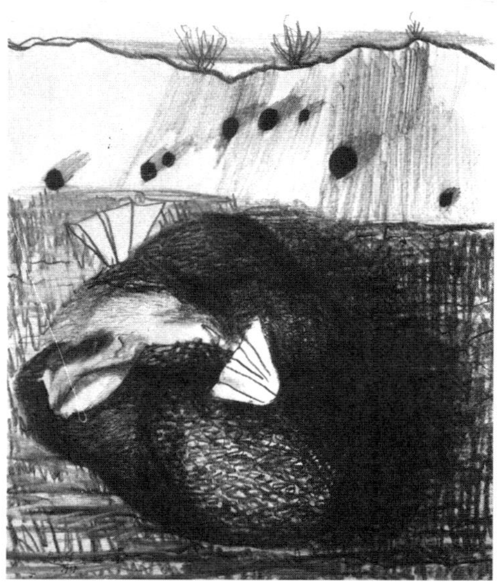

Find I, 1937, pencil and pastel on paper

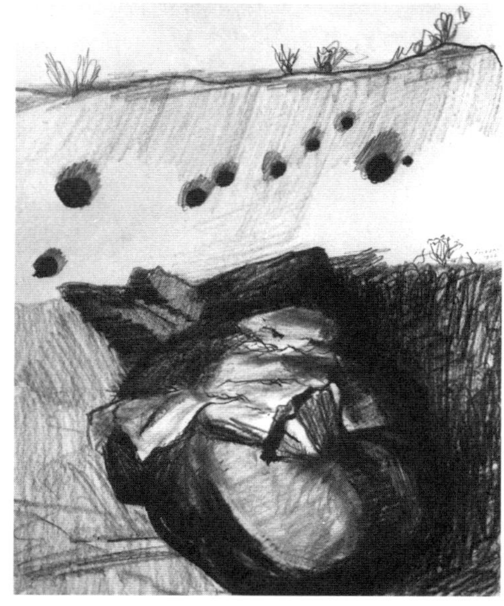

Find II, 1937, pencil and pastel on paper

XXV

Dream from the Pile

(1938)

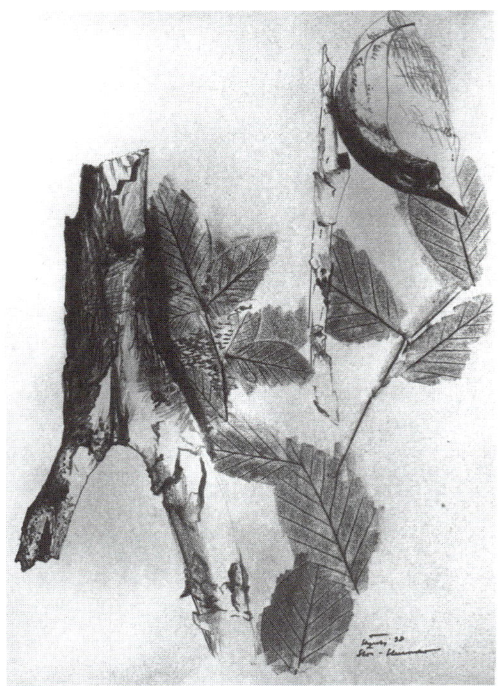

Drawing I, 1938, pencil and frottage on paper

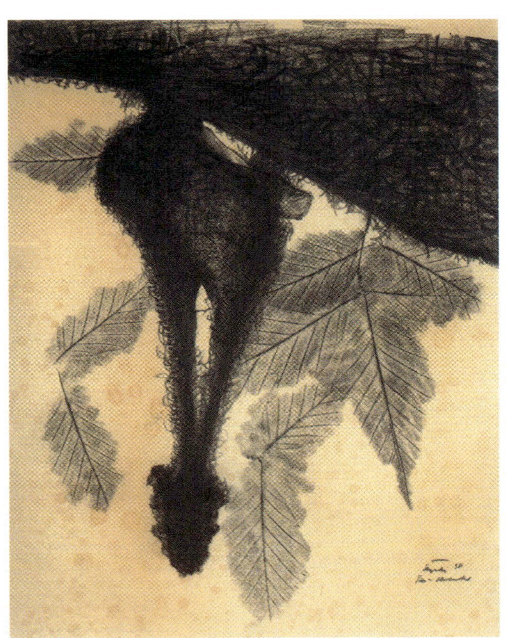

Drawing II, 1938, pencil and frottage on paper

XXVI

Dream of a Girl Frozen in Ice

(1939)

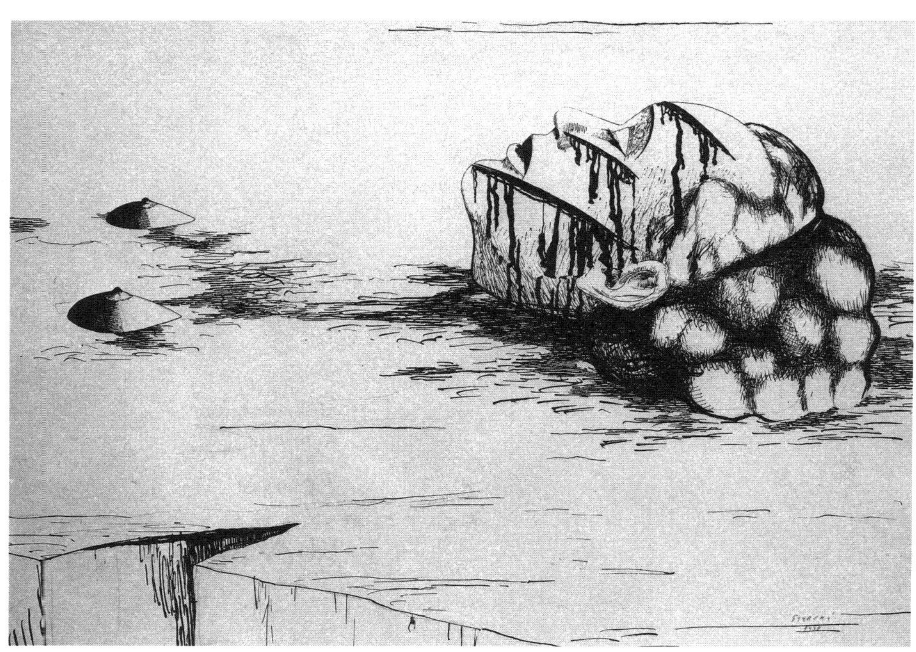

Icebound Woman I, 1939, pen and ink on paper

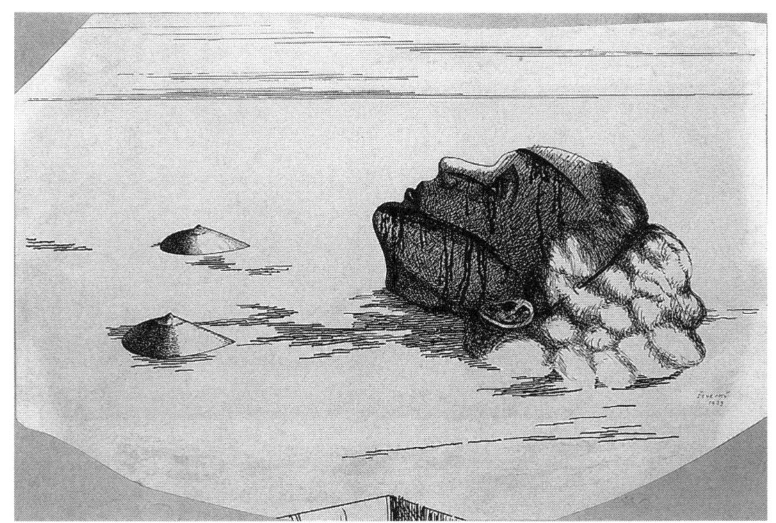

Icebound Woman II, 1939, pen and ink on paper

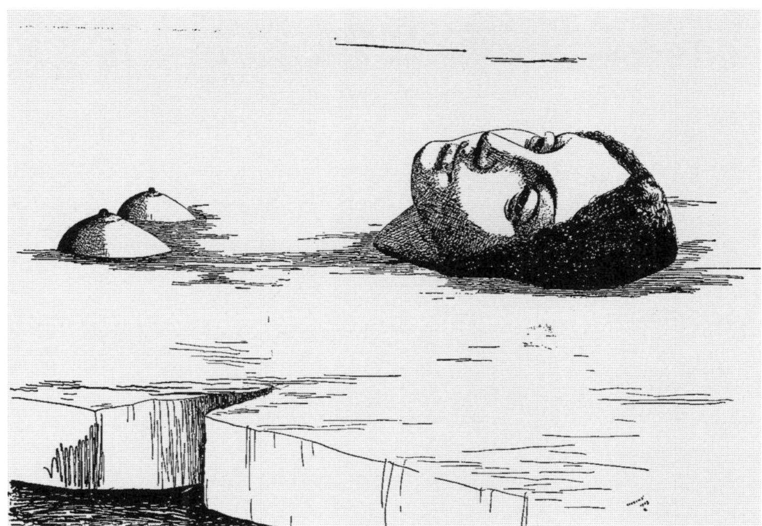

Icebound Woman III, 1939, pen and ink on paper

XXVII

Dream of Muscles

(1939)

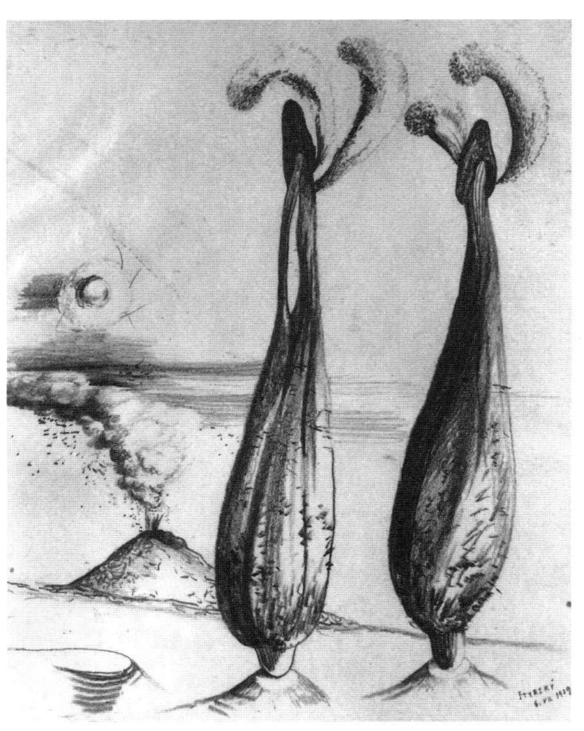

Muscles, 1939, pencil on paper

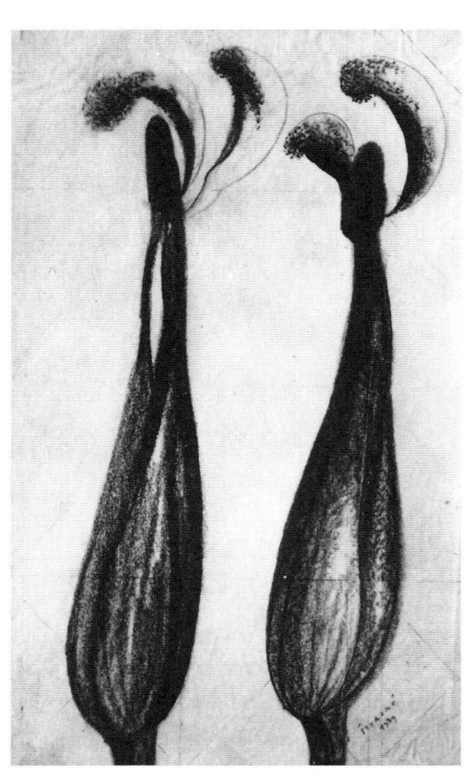

Muscles, 1939, ruddle on paper

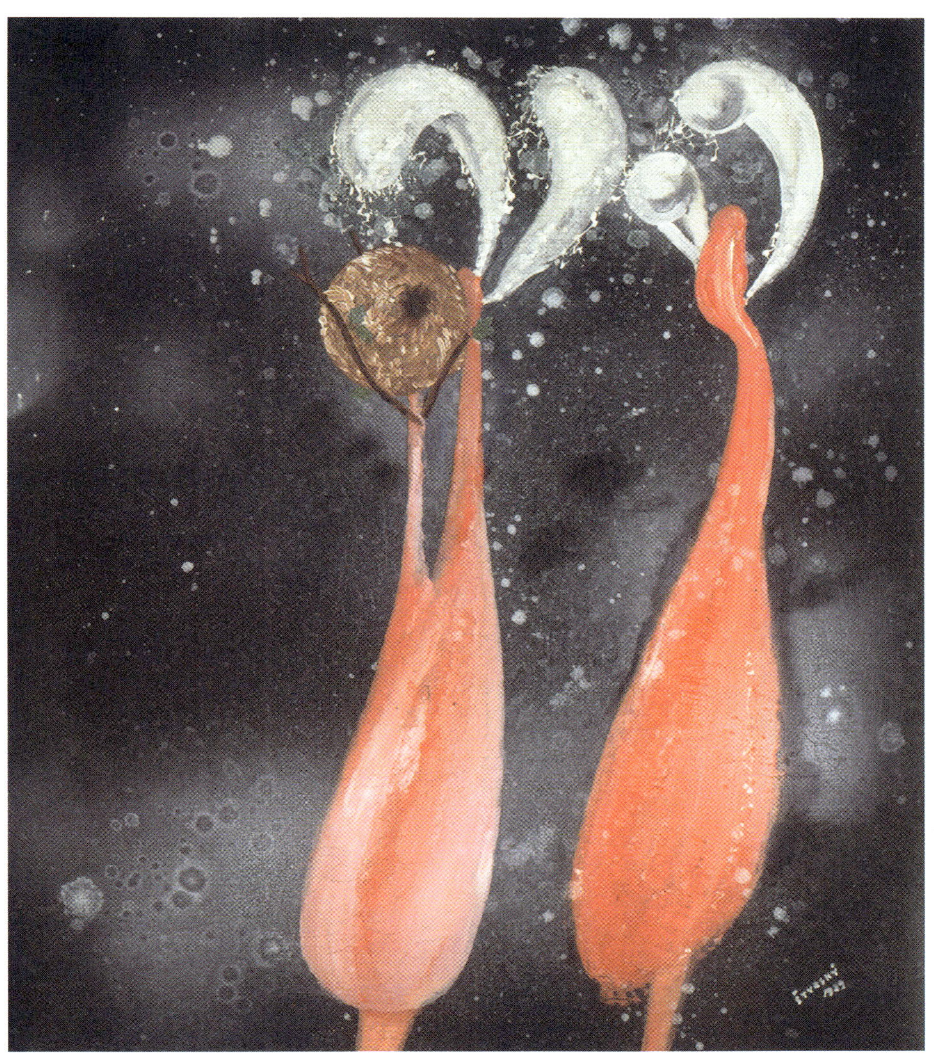

Man and Woman, 1939, oil on canvas

XXVIII

A Dream

(1939)

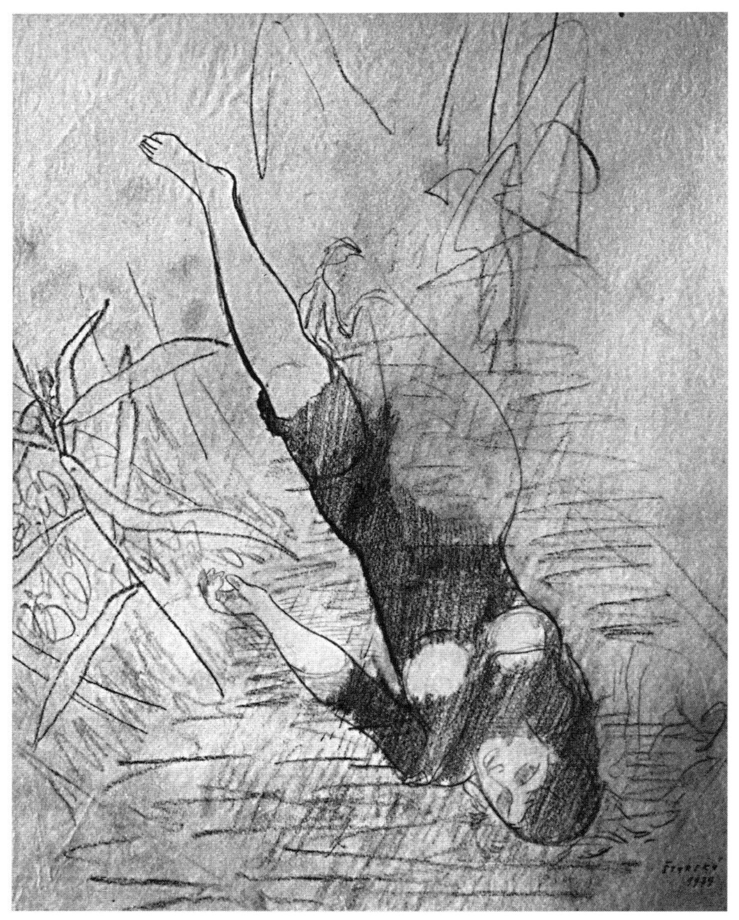

Record of Dream of Drowned Woman, 1939, pencil on paper

XXIX

Dream of the Inheritance

(THE NIGHT OF JULY 24–25, 1939)

I am walking around the garden in Čermná. Someone is calling to me that I've received an inheritance from my mother and I should go immediately to see what it is. So I go into the house, to the first floor, to the closet.* In the middle of the room stands one of those large black rustic trunks fitted with iron bands. Gleaming in its newness. I open it. It is filled with eiderdowns. I begin to straighten them out and stack them up on the floor, tables, everywhere I find a free space, but the trunk is still filled with them. The room is filled with them as well all the way to the ceiling : white pillows, striped duvets, embroidered cushions, heavy quilts, a bale of loose bedding, etc. Finally a layer of clothes appears in the trunk. They are the dresses my mother wore when I was a child, among which I recognize a violet silk dress, then an avalanche of dresses that belonged to my sister, and a floral dress I've never seen before. A bundle of lace and shawls. Then I discover the trunk has a hidden compartment full of rosaries, holy relics, various mementos from places of pilgrimage, round powder boxes, several vials of Digitalis, and two dried Roses of Jericho. Now I think I will find something truly valuable, but it's only skirts, black cotton petticoats, and a variety of bodices. Eventually I pick up a dress, and under it I uncover the life-size figure of Little Apple.** She's painted on plywood in the style of American placards, the contours of her body cut precisely to detail, and she's wearing nothing but a white

* It's a long room that for as long as I can remember served as a storage space for broken furniture, disused objects, broken vases, funeral wreaths in enormous boxes, dried wedding bouquets, bundles of newspapers, old books, discarded parasols, square hat boxes, the price tags littering the floor, old magazines, and assorted correspondence. It was a paradise for spiders and mice. It was my childhood paradise. (1941)

** The name I gave a certain girl.

chemise, panties, hose, and pink slippers on her feet. I decide to stand her up in the room because I'm infatuated with her, aroused.

— — — — it's nearly night. The room is growing dark. I sense that something has changed. When I look to a corner, I see standing there the figures of my father and mother, leaning against the wall, looking like they did in their wedding photograph : Mother dressed in white, holding a bridal bouquet, and Father wearing a long frock. Both are made of clay — the word "golem" comes to mind — and in the moonlight I see how old the clay is, cracked — — —.

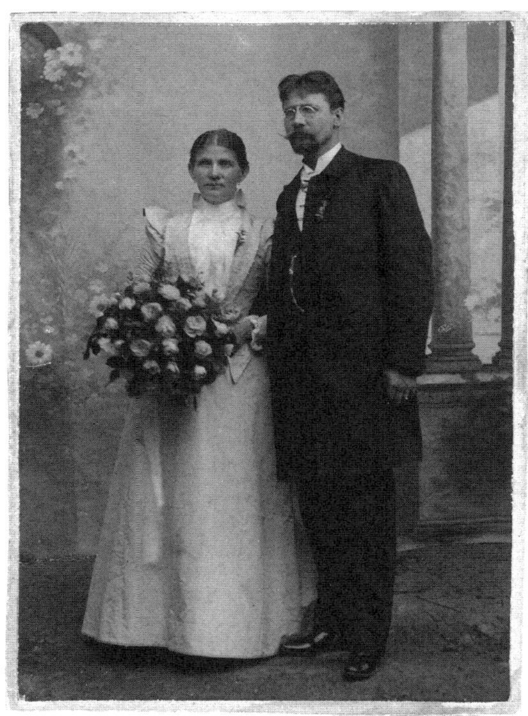

Wedding portrait of my parents

XXX

Dream of the Deserted House

(SUMMER 1940)

I am standing in front of an old derelict house built of rough stone, unplastered. The windows and door are boarded up. I walk around it to see if there might be a way in. When I've walked around three sides, I notice on the *eastern* side, where the house abuts a garden, female legs protruding from the wall. As if a woman has been immured here. A stocking and a shoe cover one leg, and the other has been picked clean to the bone. I want to get into the house. Bears. I rip one of the boards from a window and break into the house. Then I barricade the window and am satisfied I'm safe. I lie down on a bed and sleep. — — A particular noise jolts me from the dream — — — maybe it was my regular breathing. Light enters the room, and in a corner above me, above the bed, are giant cobwebs, dense, as if hundreds of years old, but instead of spiders there are two copulating frogs — — — breathing deeply — — —

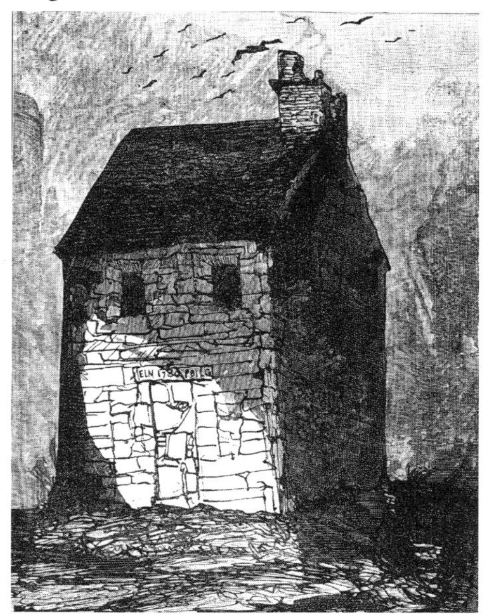

Victor Hugo's illustration *La maison visionée*

Note from 1940 : After many years, this past spring I reread Victor Hugo's *Toilers of the Sea* and compared the translation with the original edition (*Les Travailleurs de la Mer*) that included Hugo's xylograph illustrations. The source of this dream obviously is one of the illustrations : LA MAISON VISIONNÉE.

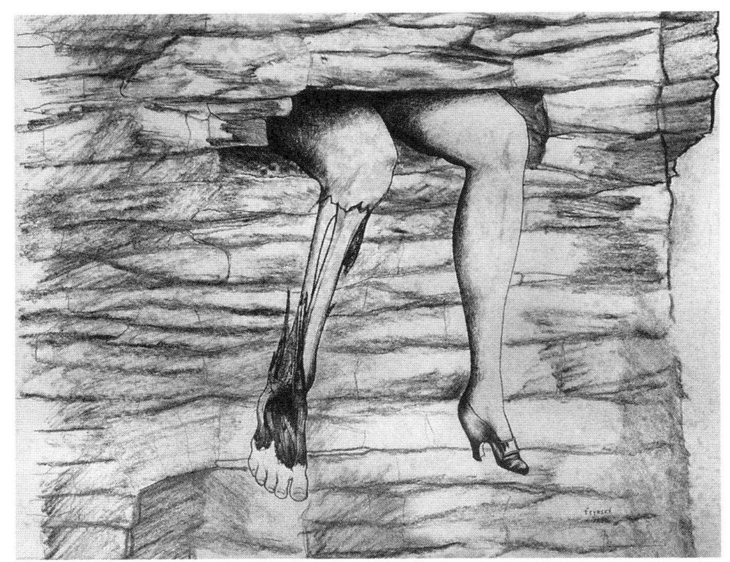

Dream of the Deserted House, 1940, pencil on paper

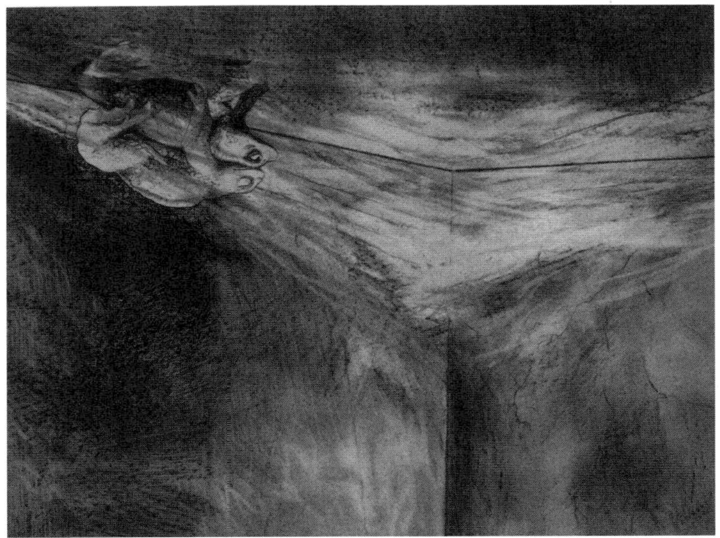

Dream of the Deserted House, 1940, pencil on paper

XXXI

Dream of the Grove in Nedošín, or, Dream of the Somnambulist's Muse

(JULY 1940)

On a sunny afternoon I am lying with Cinderella in a small clearing in the Nedošín grove (we're kissing). Cinderella is wearing nothing more than a sheer dress of white etamine (as if transparent); several times she reminds me she's not wearing underclothes (she has on white flats without socks); she looks completely white to me (magnificent long legs bared to mid-thigh); it occurs to me that she should be tanned from being out in the sun (I tell her this, and she hikes up her dress a bit further); on her crotch I discover five snails clinging to her skin and pubic hairs, and when I uncover her belly I see another stuck to her navel (and when she completely undresses for me I find another snail under her breasts and another in her armpit); I kiss her again and we make love . . .

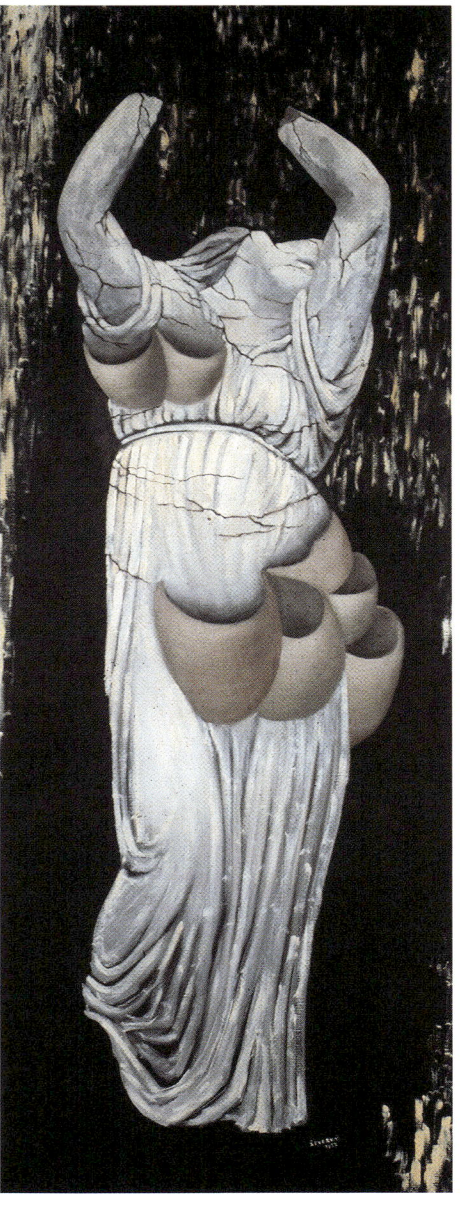

The Somnambulist's Muse, 1937, oil on canvas

XXXII

Dream of Fish

(1940)

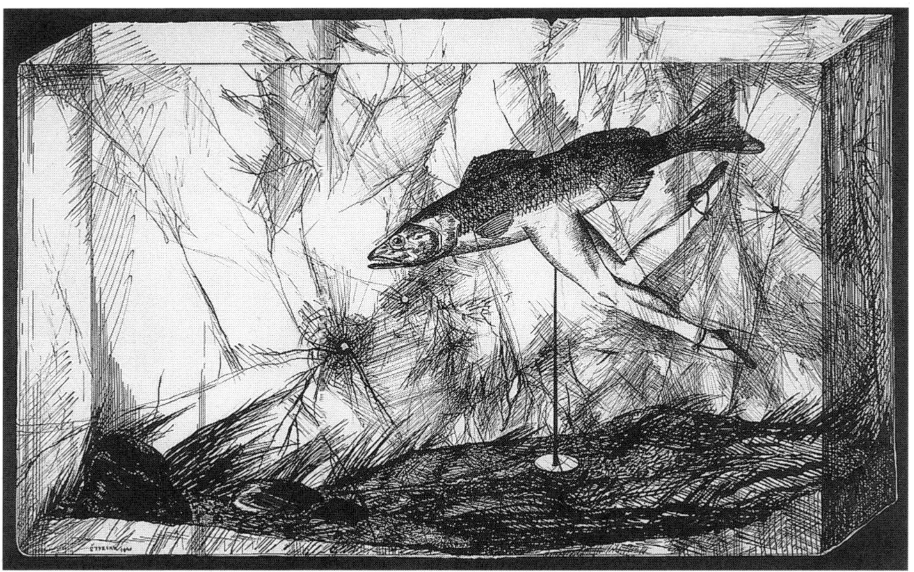

Dream of Fish I, 1940, pen and ink on paper

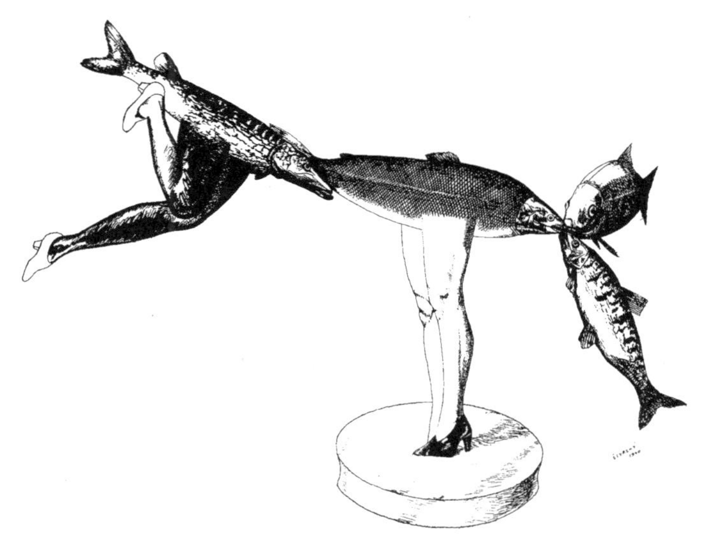

Dream of Fish II, 1940, pen and ink on paper

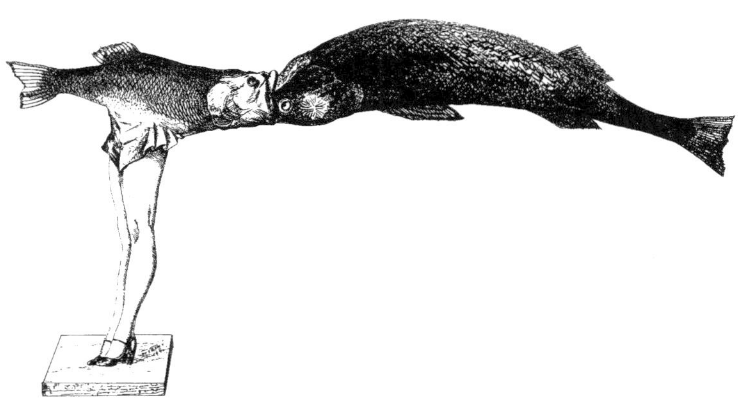

Dream of Fish III, 1940, pen and ink on paper

XXXIII

Dream of the Webbed Hand

(DECEMBER 27, 1940)

In the hall of a Viennese palace. A high chamber. Tall doors painted white, closed. The lock isn't located, as is usual, in the middle of the door, but way up by the ceiling. The doors are likely locked. Someone is trying to pick the lock from the outside. The lock falls off, and in the opening a hand appears, its fingers connected by webbing.

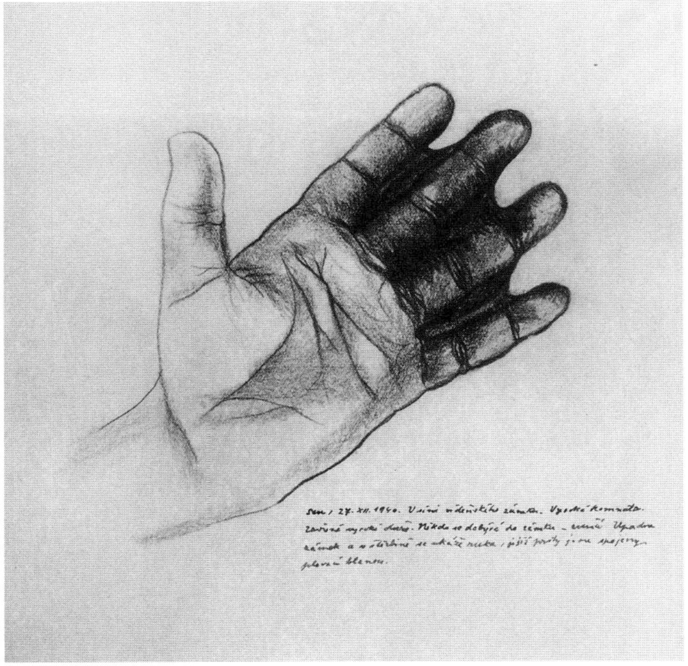

Dream Record, 1940, pencil and pastel on paper

VERSE

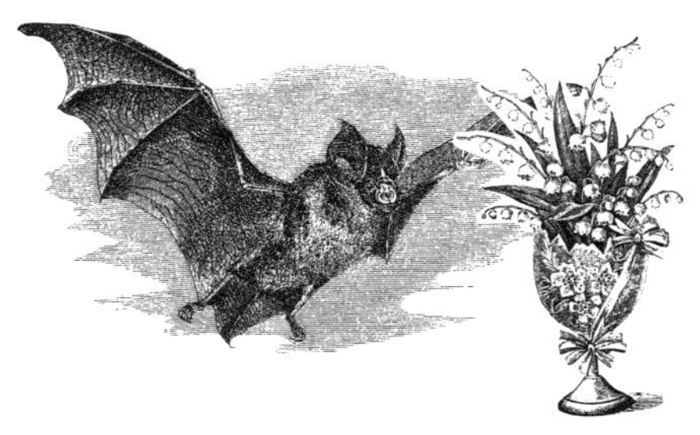

Alcohol and a Rose

Today's art is highly entertaining : Art it is not.
Life has poetry.
        Poetry is a string of nonsense.
The world is full of fine ventures, poems, paintings,
but boring (quality does not negate boring),
logical (more logic than beauty you'll notice).
Poetry itself = nonsense. In life = contrary
to the pragmatic. Necessity.
        The life we lead in our offices, families, etc.,
        save the time we spend with lovers,
        bores us.
                We need adventure.
The life of adventure ends under the watchful eye
of Dr. Heveroch.
                We need pragmatic intellect.
We consume poetry like poison (arsenic).
Art does not weigh on our heart like a stone, like a sweet
        burden.
                We live.
We have poetry : of sunsets,
        of tourism (restaurants at castle ruins),
        (motorhomes),
        of sport (scout nymphs),
        of bars and dances (exchange work clothes for elegant
                evening dress),
        of alcohol, adventure,
        of loves and flirtations,

of French cuisine.
Of history as lovely as a modern painting
(not factual of course),
of cinema, movie stars,
of circuses, the cabaret,
of outings, parks,
of absolute absurdity,
of books of poetry,
of books of pictures.
Art has never had a patent on beauty,
and poetry never will.
Let's not make from our lives poetry,
let's not make professional poetry,
but let's not deprive ourselves of poetry.
Yesterday needed art to stave off exhaustion,
Today needs poetry to enjoy life.
And I need,
as long as it's needed,
alcohol,
a rose,
forgotten in a public toilet.

Cemetery 1923

A stone angel cannot count
Rosy mounds of soil
Tender words shudder
On gilded inscriptions
Translucent smiles
Memories
Slender stalks of lilies
Words immobilized in a scented breeze
Bluebell eyes
A kiss sucks out the death rotting in a breast

Rumlights

Death on machine peripheries
Forgotten tombs
Pale arbors inviting entry
Houses like impregnable safes
A key

Young women hair freshly waved
Color running at the first rain
Ageless harpies
Greek simians
Papuans
Abyssinians
And the so-called other elite
A staircase of spiritists
And an outcry over paid seats evoking *Das Rhinegold*

I meant to offer this charmed circle
assistance

No Cherries, Birds, Nets Here

Earth
Tract
Curve

Without season
Without rain
Tireless for eternity

Odd orchid clusters
Chests clenched in pain
Their jaws injurious
Green tubes fanning out
And devouring light

Roots rampant in these bizarre conditions
In the light
While night encloses the crowns of olive trees

Yet day merges with it
Always the same

Rosy
The form of a cog railway
Fabricated with precision
Stopping on a whim
Discharging occasional waterfalls

Flowing
Multicolored

Packs of women
With heads like snowballs
With eyes and mouths of diverse construct
Protruding
Like mountain tops blooming with gentians

Sugarbowl Saltceller & Pepperbox

To shake the petals off Carlsbad roses
Growth in furry catkins

On abandoned verandas
The fallen leaves of autumn tablecloths
Green chairs

Prophetic madness
Makes another appearance behind the door
Leading into the room filled half with pepper
Half with salt

And at times even the pond shadows mirror illusory movement

Calumniating one another
Their mutual respect intact
This is the life of reeds mire and fish
Not for man's disdain

The Blind Medium in the Louvre

Cecilia Cecilia
Don't drink the toxic water
Caw caw caw

Hypnotized by her wreckage
Memory!
Proof
In multiple mirrors
Caw caw
Memory!
Proof
Dew falls
Tea-colored
Of lemons
Cecilia caw caw
Proof proof
Tea-colored
Of lemons
Toxic water
Proof Cecilia

Only Night

Only night can disorient a child
Concealing his first stiff collar
In which he has sinned

Becoming a rooster
In a ballet that starts
Without wasting time on crowing

This mount of emotions
Stacked like flapjacks
Listless and static
Sunken by the weight

Leaves of Ice

I scared the parrots from their crests
The vulgar colors of memories paling
And a green peacock proudly
Crying and wailing in the branches

The looted crypts of its eyes
An endless keyboard monotoned
The rotting nerves of its eyes
In eternal blackness
And colorless
The eyes of blind smokers
Wielding intoxicating woodbeams

I Looked for Ash in Ash

Rosebush amid the lawn

I wanted to be a circus equestrienne

I saw you dance atop the horses
A dress of blue stars
While the lions kept roaring
Your leotard melding with the horse's back
I walked across peaks
Of ash mountains
Sinking into them

The Gang of Fake Convicts

Black dogs run in ditches
Celebrations of autumn's return
At night
People bear strange figures
And pulverize cathedrals
A gang with pickaxes and sacks of dynamite
Clamber on the portals and chip off the flowers
And marble heads

Finally a ship
Steams its way into port
The tide
The dancing skirt lace
The plump flower of a water lily
And a chubby belle

To You I Open the Five Leaves of the World

In the dark just her white dress cried for help
Yet even this vanished

Porcelain skies

At first four marching elephants
A white blizzard
3 kings came as phantoms
Camel hoofprints

Then came the landscapes of sand and white towers
Stone books
Gardens of metal roses
And small tea-colored Klára

The Strange Death of the Butcher's Wife in District X

Blue night distant
To where we hasten

An auto's bugling
All there is

Though we are able
To listen to hairless creatures
Stroking the skin of a frog
Is beyond us

Not Arnoštka not the sanguine countryside
Can move someone used to tenderness
Governed by his moods
For instance
Spitting under chairs
Occupied by those
Who should be sitting
On Arnoštka's hat

In the Swamps

The fortune of blackcaps flies over the surface
In the guise of moorhens ripe for a dawn shooting
By passionate hunters and hedonists

A wounded bird falls to the dead surface
Arms of brunettes pulling it down

At times they emerge above the water
Bitten by the jaws of hounds

Then a horde of black swine
Their snouts rooting
Sodden sacks of gold
While a man on a pedestal
Speaks

I Built a Box

I built a box
Verdigris
Stalks
An aquarium, into it I threw Marie's glove
To always have in my sight
The ruin

Dead verdigris
Dead stalks
And the broken handle of a parasol
Dead moons
Of moss
A celluloid nymph gone soft

Many strange creatures
Were not born in water

The Soporific Speak

He lives without successor

Massive breasts and holidays
In these ruins
Trees have leaves
The color of ink

Sleeping at last
Sleeping on a bee hand
Far from the wellsprings of sleep

Acetic thoughts circle
A respectable life
Clear in their logic

If My Speech Were a Torrent of Four Flows

I have known three types of satiation
The pitch a raven cannot hit
A hutch where a swine plays the dandy
Burial mounds not built from curses

I was to be the owner of vast stables with maiden jockeys

And immense black-and-white plantations
Where queenless pawns
Undermine my authority

I'm still waiting
For mills to churn cacti
And they will turn
Beguiling the prickly and the powdered
Under the mountains

Do You Hear the End Bells?

I was caught unawares
When the monster of Kateřina took possession of me

She swam against the current of my sleep

While she rode my body
Proudly erect like in the saddle
I envisaged the
Peerless envoy of my desires

A white path led from my door

Only Harps Now Love Silence

A toad sleeping on a clock
A clock showing toad time

Everything happens under turbid water
Where maidens sit reading
Under green water
Luckily
Coats of their own skin
Made whenever we wish

Expensive skin

But when the eye of God looks on us toads
It'll take delight
In we toads clad in the fur of divine mice
Theirs is the Kingdom of Heaven

Emilie Liked to Undress

Acacias of smoke

Stale talk
How else to explain the swallowing of tears

If only I could remember those days
Leaves falling into baskets
Pipes
Lakes
Hats

Only Emilie's plaid dress
Made leaving Pavlína so easy
A creature of night going down to the bawdyhouses
Behind the cascades of a Chinese pavilion
In a yellow dress
Long calves

Jeannette vanished
A cube of low-grade margarine was all of her that remained

I couldn't call Pavlína a pearl
And still I paid dearly for her roots

Don't let her aloofness fool you
This pale girl with husky eyes
Marguerite de Navarre

And all the anonymous nymphs of this century
Live in peace
Like golden lilies fading in the sun
My sole adventure
A full beard

Solveig

Solveig has five hearts
The fifth coated in hair
And blind

Musk
The ticklish sweat of cat hair
That has slept in a bed of lilies
With laundry-room odor

I walked slowly
My head at the hem of her skirt

I saw her skin show through
And the hairs on her calves
Disheveled beneath her stockings
I wanted to straighten them
Imagining the type of comb required

Solveig then sauntered
Like a gummy green baboon
The fallen leaves of autumn
Sticking to her

Stone

Stone is evil
Brick is not stone
Only when old brick breaks up
Then is it stone

Giant rock terraces retain heat
And caves the cold
Rocks deepened by the sun
Shaping chasms and wells
(Like a piece of meat well roasted)

These hollows extend into the rocks' depths
Where they meet with cold
That pushes them deeper

In a villa's verdure
Distant
A cube with balconies of plaited lattice
Girls in white dresses flit behind

The stars wattle marble tablets
And at night a lit skyscraper
Floats in the sea

Fatigue

Sand will drift
Over the paths taken by Pavlína
That will be called error
No one will manage to fathom
Or even explain

Except the autumn evenings
And despair
Nothing here deserving a sheet of paper

Love's techniques are always varied

You'll be the world's most exquisite ruin

The Ever-Shrinking World

I imagine a girl's movement, I dissect horror and memory, and nothing from the sacks of silliness I sit on escapes me.

Emilie with the tiny Chinese feet is dead. I save only one lamp without stars, an orb without light. A mirror without image, ruins without memories. In the ivy and in that dwarf nut I rediscovered history, drawn out and losing itself in the melancholy of youth's bloom, entangled in the memories of days past.

Broken youth floats in houses, houses float in bedrooms, bedrooms float in linen closets, and all of it bathed in light.

Amid the thicket of black crosses, sunken graves, a moss-covered photograph on enamel, wreaths of glass pearls, vases with yellowed putrefying water like custard, a tissue forming stalks of lace interwoven with vines of ivy. Hanging over the wall from the neighboring garden is a small branch with two oranges. Hooked nails, snail shells, coral scattered in clay, a harvestman peregrinating rusted wires.

I would like to paint your portrait into the midst of this cemetery scenery, the face of my sea woman, her image engraved on a flaking wall, fissured, soaked by rain, saturated with water, chapped by a windstorm, ravaged by time. Several dried flowers placed between books by a sylphic hand and a fading photograph, these are the only mementos left to me.

I saw the evening star rise over the ruins, the path becoming lost in the creeping undergrowth and ultimately in the thicket of carnivorous plants. First cockcrow. Morning star. Hands, your amazing hands, turning black as coal. When I stepped on them they disintegrated into mush and mire. And yet, I remember remarkably little of my youth.

I recall a coffin that stood in my grandmother's attic. She kept apples in it, until she was put there herself. The coffin smelled like apple. The rays of autumn sun always penetrated the squares of window at two p.m. without marring the casket's silver fittings. No discoloration, no turning green.

A spring landscape, standing against the wind, the wind forming a cast of her bosom and legs. Clothed in a light white dress and white slippers, she stands at the iron railing, a pattern of regular spirals.

The group ate, swaying in the wind, memories of past lives, a painter of remote walls in Provence, a painter of spilled blood. The silence of mute eyes, the silence of wounds gaping and powdered, the silence of worn walls.

Two doves rose into a pale blue sky.

Water rushing through the houses, splashing and overflowing the chimneys, chairs floating in the barren wasteland of water, pictures among the carcasses of sheep and sweaters. One's native region is always boring and monotonous.

My feet have drowned in the pavement. Hair has fallen in a mane from the cliffs. Eve dances in the middle of the street, her face lit by a cigarette. The first drops of alcohol accumulate in vegetal wombs. Time for the first knife and the first wind harp.

I was wearing lingerie that was too long and Klára's stockings. While she believed she was married to a field marshal and slept with her hands clasped under her head on the gravestone, three monkeys washed her feet, obstructed by a muscular brute kneeling before her, his head on her knee. But they paid him no mind as they scrubbed her lovely calf until the flesh fell from it, forming a morass of blood.

Flying gemstones and in the caves a wind harasses the tongues of forgotten fires.

Red hummingbirds selecting their spots in dazzling fiery green, blue ostriches finding yellow plains of sand and crows a land of snow. Only the gray bat merges with the blue of night.

Olive and cherry trees with torn lace. Oh, tell me all about Astolaine! Astolaine, this decay of buried corpses. Astolaine, this mountain of flies, reduced by wind and turned by rain into sun-dried dough. It is tissue forming succulent stalks of lace. It is an autumnal woman with crimson hair. I called her LITTLE APPLE. I should've called her PRALINE.

I saw her in an enormous vat filled with vinegar, a thick cork around her neck. A procession of firemen with charters hanging from their mouths filed past. Then she danced in a block of thick fog. To me she seemed without contour, her figure merely a vibration of form illumined by flashes of blue light.

She came to me after the storm. I saw her kneel into ferns flecked with dew. I know each one of her eyelashes and her virtually invisible hands, I know the heavy scent of her abundant copper hair. I saw her face the shimmering woods, nude in the middle of her room. Her laughter like alabaster snowflakes, she cried over the futile embrace. I know her solitude and her selfish, precipitous heart.

I know her voice — it's edgy, tired and pure, hesitant, accusatory and callous, velvety, cold and sluggish, turbid and self-seeking. I know its depths, its glow, indifference, vindictiveness, mendacity, and vanity. I know its strength and its vertigo, its sighs, pride, and darkness. I know her voice, suppurating, wandering, silken and clanging. I know her flute-like whisper and her passivity. I also know her silence and the moment of surrender, her cries, violent explosions, her husky hostility. I heard her voice, it sounded like an organ, like the lifeless voice of old women, like the glassy voice of phantoms. I know her tinny voice, as if a contrast between dreaming and vulgarity. I know her voice that speaks and sings in a dream, her voice coming from an immense distance. IN THE END I FOUND THIS VOICE TEDIOUS.

My rusty rose! Your love was as fragrant as a late garden.

I left you for a moonlit landscape. And as I walked the landscape became transformed. I walked through hoarfrost and then on a snowy trail toward white woods. The trees were weighted with snow, and a hare was gnawing at the bark of young rowans. The trail rose through the woods, and I walked a long time, the forest beginning to thin and the snow recede. I heard the occasional twitter of a bird. I stepped on a tuft of snowdrops, walked through a meadow covered in cowslips, and stopped at a pool whose surface was silently ablaze in the sun. Only a metallic dragonfly quivered over the water. Then the leaves yellowed and Indian summer spread over the fields of stubble. I walked farther, always toward the horizon, until I finally stopped and for the first time had the clear realization that I had passed through my time as if in a dream.

On your hot miniature breasts, which I love about you most, I place a leaf to cover you with my love and to encumber you like a tombstone.

I no longer see the landscape, and you lift your eyes. Mirrors surround you, waiting for you to enter. Everything around you is submerged in artificial shadows.

They await you. Somewhere nearby you will find a key that opens this valise. To hear, feel, touch is to remember. You will touch the fern lying in wait for you each morning in the mirror. It will be cold.

Astolaine will walk around me to tread further the lawn of rhymes, assonances, and puns to the tempo of an operetta ditty. Her fate is to be a small tallow candle, or a bit larger.

For me flowers exist only by their names.

Only a dahlia had the color of skin torn from the back on a beach. Only it had the color of powder shaken from the ivy. Peonies conceal tears of water among their petals, as do all dense flowers. A gilded flower, similar to Goldband Lilies. White magnolias command silence by their presence as loud talk causes their petals to fall. Red Pyrenean forget-me-nots are like the eyes of a swan, and Normandy salad resembles green lace that has decayed and grown moldy in catacombs, crypts, and on tombs.

Sea-colored water in a glass cube, a star lying on its sandy bottom. The lawns outside my windows release green aniline during a rainstorm. It runs down the slope into the lake.

I will never again bring a sprig of almond.

Never again will I see the nocturnal procession during a lightning storm, the dolphins, bowers of rose, butterflies, lizards, bats in the cliffs, the flight of gulls over the sea, monks in cream habits and black cloaks, pines, the flight of wimples in the wind, and women on rose balconies amid flowerpots.

Fossilized heart, fossilized memories, fossilized books, fossilized stars, fossilized lampblacks, fossilized cheeses, fossilized wrinkles, fossilized velvet, fossilized graves.

One day a band of Ahasueruses will come and peel off the dirt and clean your garments, then they will again spin their tops on the road and continue on their way.

Fossilized sky, fossilized dreams, fossilized lakes. Lakes suggest death. Above lakes, woods are impotent solace.

Fragments

Nudity shrouded in cigar smoke — sweet hills.

A dirty drunk, but his collar is clean.

A girl coalesced with a balustrade.

Phantoms — coquettes and barrels of black coffee.

Red furnaces — ovens — when all the steel goes white, snow falls.

Spring : floral slippers.

On the ice at St. Moritz : shadows shifting, individuals effaced.

Fog — gray sea and gray sky. A gray silhouette in the distance slowly emerging from the fog; only when it approaches can the young boy be recognized as gray.

David and Miss Goliath.

A Lowood swan with a neck of stovepipe.

He made love like a chainsaw.

Mask in a tree. A tree of ripening masks.

A lovely young girl leading a military band.

Dance is the taming of females.

A young girl assaulted and groaning under the weight of a rapturous beast.

Dog snout in the grass.

Roads are tree branches placed along the ground.

Cathedrals of bird feathers.

Blondes look good with white cones in their mouths.

The vampire is a sweetheart, his energy gently waning from his lack of prejudice. One does not befriend a vampire, only loves him before he starts to bore.

Paradise in the hues of cholera and plague.

Leaves create more than the tree, for example, a bouquet, an elephant, or a silly-looking hat can be made from them.

The whisper of combs.

The tropics — a butterfly collection beneath a zebra's dugs.

Sunsets over cucumber salads.

The sculpture of a woman, bent over and balancing in the wind. This is the winter that has passed.

The harbor is strange at night, the gates closed, only the sea's portals operate on their own, and the slight figure of a lighthouse, the harbor front deserted and dimly lit. There is nothing more mysterious than mute forms.

An onyx figurine, blood flowing through its veining.

The heart of the upper lip suggests chaste, old-world belles, while the lower lip, accustomed to being kissed, conjures up images of whorehouse flora.

We've struck vice and sin from our vocabulary.

Grape clusters of eyes.

Sandstone figures in a room (Mother and Father).

Horse in the cathedral (I lead the horse away from Mass).

On the grave grow pumpkins and tomatoes.

Landscapes from my rumpled bed (quilts). Spring in my bed.

A carp with a lady's dainty legs.

A girl from the 1870s in a carboniferous forest.

A bed with a corpse in a garden by the sea.

WRITINGS

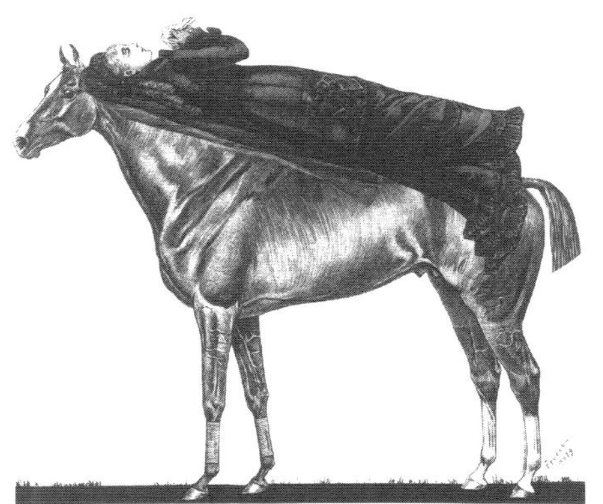

From a Lecture at Masaryk University in Brno

Out of necessity, modern painting has freed itself of its narrative function, its epic and genre character without giving up its dramatic nature. It has converted its outmoded, literary dramatic nature into the drama of form, line, color, and material. It excludes everything impressionistic and illusionistic while the photographic image excludes so-called art photography. As such, painting and photography take on a purity of expression and legitimate one another without being rivals.

•

Painting is the poetry of sight. It has no other purpose than to be poetry. And this is its social utility. The painting is a poetic vision of the world. The painting could never be realistic even though it might be created from reality, from the elements of reality. It could never truck in illusionism, because a concrete lyrical vision is woven into its web of abstraction. It is neither window nor display case (Derain). It is a magical surface, which despite all its concrete aspects remains a surface.

•

Poetry has no need of logic, just as beauty has no need of logic. Yet to create a poetic painting requires intellectual rigor and diligence. The art of today contains much that is illogical ordered by logic. The raison d'être of painting surely is not to be understood. Since it is delight, art is in no way rational, and if delight were rational it would be boring. Emotion in contemporary art is purely physiological and affective, not psychological. The profundity of the modern human does not lie hidden in the depths of the soul but on the surface, overt, transparent, self-evident. The painting solves no problems; it does not edify, nor, importantly, does it teach character — this is not its function.

A painting's form determines a particular sensation in people that stimulates mental images, analogies of images, connecting waves, or the modern painter's methods are more complex, and he groups together myriad images inspired by a particular object that does not even appear in the painting, and these visions facilitate other visions in viewers, ultimately a vision of their primal origin.

•

Who knows, maybe on May 1 we will issue a manifesto that art is once again art, not in the sense of a return but as something entirely new. Ilya Ehrenburg felt a need to exclaim : "Art has stopped being art." He was stating the obvious. Art had indeed stopped being art. We needed time to sort out the luggage we call art, luggage needed for a pleasant journey through life. We've thrown out the old and obsolete and furnished ourselves with much that's indispensable. Of course, we could take the journey without this luggage, and admittedly it would lighten our load, though we would always feel as if something were missing, something were wanting. It would be a little idiotic to renounce what isn't a burden when nothing is lost by holding onto it.

A Popular Introduction to Artificialism

Though Pythagoras was the first to construct a necklace he forgot the harlots

we are proclaiming artificialism in painting without any ambition to outfit the rabble with magical glasses to view the world with in order to find their place in it

artificialism initiates a new era for painting that will be dated to the two faces of janus identifying with one another thanks to which the herd will never stomp through it

we are modern to the extent we're not sure if we're contemporary

we have retained a single innocence the mirror without image artificialism will not be an epidemic like dada etc.

only the real is absurd the future of painting assured by a nun who crossed its path if flowers fell off in autumn what would the leaves do

artificialism is an adventure whose ending is unknowable and the only way to avoid it is by losing it

artificialism has no graves so no one can ever bring it flowers

we have loved this assortment of seconds but it became ossified while we were thinking about it

and while you become acclimated to your ideas of artificialism you will either love or howl only at illusion

pleas and invectives will be impotent

artificialism is the gravedigger of your idiocy

there is no reason to attach importance to anything in this text

it matters very little to us if you deteriorate by old age or paralysis others shall bring us joy

artificialism creates no uniformity

why should you protest against or sympathize with artificialism it's pointless to do so it will still be here when you're gone

Lesson I. insatiate abuse is proof of immortality

Lesson II. we will not be held accountable for artificialism's consequences

artificialism is a zone where firemen always arrive too late

to erect an artificial venus nearby security guards are needed

solace eventually every one of you degenerates

we thought up artificialism as we had nothing else to do and we never thought to dance on the head of this fury

if only we would've found a nest of hardboiled eggs somewhere

artificialism is not a society for the like- and unlike-minded

painting traversed the world like angels cherub and moccasin only to scalp folks paw fruit snap trees and stare at the countryside

merdre merdre merdre[1]

epilogue the last lines lapse into indolence blurring the final remnants of reflections we might still inflict from a lack of consciousness of what we call life

Štyrský & Toyen

[1] The modified spelling of *merde* [shit] that begins Alfred Jarry's play *Ubu Roi*.

Artificialism

Cubism was a product of traditional painting, which divided painting into figurative, landscape, and still life with varying degrees of descriptiveness. At root this was a new method and technique of representation. It replaced trompe l'oeil with the illusion of reality spatially disseminated. It generally viewed the painting through the prism of a model. Pictorial forms coincided with real forms, and where this proved impossible it gave way to distortion. Dissecting reality resulted in mirroring and duplication. Rather than activate the imagination, Cubism skewed reality. When it had achieved maximum reality, it discovered it had no wings. Eyes that had gradually become sensitive continually squinted at the horizon of their origin, so what ensued was an illogical return to "nature." Even so, Cubism gave painting *unlimited possibilities.*

Artificialism has an inverse perspective. Leaving reality alone, it *strives for a maximum of imagination.* By not manipulating reality it can continue to delight in it, having no ambition to equate a clown's cap to a geometric solid, which has no other allure than as infallible abstraction, yet this is enough to satisfy poets conversant with mystification. A mirror without image. Artificialism *identifies the painter with the poet.*[2] It repudiates painting as merely a play of form and eye candy (nonfigurative art). It repudiates figurative historicism in painting (Surrealism). Artificialism has an abstract awareness of reality. It does not deny the existence of reality, but does not work with it. Its sole focus is POETRY, which fills the gaps between real forms and emanates from reality. It responds to the poetry latent within real forms with a positive continuity. Exteriority is a function of the poetic perception of memory (negative continuity). Of memory of memories. Imagination loses connection to the real. The inference of memories without recourse to remembrance and experience constitutes a conception of painting whose quintessence and condensation automatically preclude any form of mirroring, thus situating memories in imaginary spaces.

[2] Cf. Karel Teige, "Malířství a poezie" [Painting and Poetry], *Disk* 1 (May 1923), 19-20 and "Manifest poetismu" [Manifesto of Poetism], *ReD* vol. 1, no. 9 (June 1928).

Memory is an extension of perception. If perceptions are transfigured at inception, then memories become abstract. They are the result of a conscious choice, a rejection of fantasy, and they pass through consciousness without either leaving a mark or fading.

Abstract visual memories at the stage of diffusion result in new formations that have nothing in common with reality or with artificial nature. This stage does not coincide with the receptive and passive state of artificial paradises nor with the aleatory logic of freaks.

The function of the intellect is extrinsic and finite. It organizes and disciplines and to an extent burnishes the vehement expressions of emotion. The process of *identifying the painter with the poet* is intrinsic, indivisible, and simultaneous.

The Artificialist painting is not bound to reality under conditions of time, locus, and space, therefore it does not lend itself to associative visions. Reality and the forms of the painting repel one another. The greater their relative distance, the more visually dramatic the emotive charge, giving rise to analogies of emotion, connective ripples, reverberations always more distant and complex, so that reality and the picture seem utterly incompatible with one another in any confrontation between them.

The Artificialist painting radiates poetic emotion beyond the optical and excites sensibilities beyond the visual. It diverts viewers from the carousel of their customary imagination, demolishing the system and mechanism of coherent ideas. Artificialism abstracts from real spaces. What emerges is a universal space, often replaced by surface distances, thereby forms are contingent on distance. Color itself has already been subjected to the effects of light, thus any anomaly of diffuse and condensed light has no impact. Lyrical ambience is created by color value and transposition.

The composition of a painting, having arisen out of a disinterest in reality, assumes total awareness and is contingent on the concrete logic of the Artficialist painting. It is absolutely definitive, immutable, and static. Forms in the painting coincide with eidetic memory. The title given the painting is neither caption nor thematic appellation but is indicative of its character and a directive for emotion. Theme and the painting are one. Its forms are self-explanatory.

Štyrský & Toyen

Three Chapters from a Book in Progress

IV

CRUSADE AGAINST THOSE WE'VE LOVED

HYGIENE OF MEMORIES

regarding cubism we're not talking about bedbugs picasso gave painting unlimited possibilities the fateful chance of which only a memory remains regarding picasso we're conversing with a memory leapfrogging eras

PARADISE IN ASHES

let's not forget those enchanting autos-da-fé on piazza della signoria where girolamo savonarola[3] with great élan arranged a nature morte from cards flacons mirrors ultimately on the strings of the mask of arlechin and shirted pulcinella

KALEIDOSCOPE OF DISGUISES

charm's waning refinement in 1907 the African sculpture barbaric eyes growing sensitive while squinting at the horizon of its origin thus picasso arrived at the zaftig muses of a return to nature

DISAPPOINTMENT

it seemed this squinting eye would emit jets of water though we've found the repertoire of the peripatetic performers of convention a meager table endlessly repeating discredited practices conscious of the primal connectedness of things hence cubism is a bricked-up window a balance of traditional painting divided into figurative landscape and still life with varying degrees of descriptiveness

DITTO

picasso never found a ballerina sleeping in an apricot still life his sorcery from the outset exhausted itself in his role as solver of given equations a cross to which we nail the robbed innocent

[3] A Dominican friar (1452–98) known for his pious "bonfire of the vanities" who defied the pope and was subsequently hanged and burned in Florence's main square.

INFIDELITY OF TONGUES

the dutch painted still lifes to stimulate appetite for food the cubists from a lack of imagination which nevertheless gave us some enjoyment until we realized this fruit was picked over dregs

POSH INTERIORS

traditional and impressionist painting made the image a window post-impressionists a display case and picasso plowed parquet

GEOMETRY AND A COMPASS

innocence prevented picasso from using these charms he was born in a land of shame

AGAINST TOURISM

picasso had difficulty scaling the highest mountains of the world when he stood on the summit he discovered he had no wings

SHAMELESSLY

he deloused painting which had become boring he disinfected the ateliers which we call cowsheds he gifted to the world a guitar and read in the cards the fortune of film we were not chummy with constructivists and bedbugs in our youth

XI

AS THE AVANT-GARDE LACKS IN ABSURDITY

IT SO LACKS IN REALITY

AXIOM

QUALITY MODERNISM

QUALITY MODERNISM

QUALITY MODERNISM

SCHOOL FOR ADVENTURERS

we scorn history avant-gardes cathedrals and those who knock out their windows with stones revolutions as barricades always resemble tombs eternal truths as they are so tedious that we have taken lies for truth and have piled them into a cone out of which the marvelous spills

TWO PARALLELS

at a time when the avant-garde is screaming for photography and film to supplant painting we have replaced both with MYSTIFICATION THE MODERN PAINTER WILL BEAR BUDS NOT FRUIT

FOUR DOG HEADS

are more beautiful than chaplin's eyes our paintings are a feast for the eye as long as these eyes do not belong to grazing cattle

WE DEMONSTRATE NEW PAINTING
AS A JUGGLING OF VISUAL
FORMS AND ANTI-OPIATE
ARTIFICIALISM
BEFORE THIS SPELL UNIVERSALIZES IT WEARS OFF

XIII

OUR REPERTOIRE

we've made a toy in the form of a ring of saturn on which wax maenads gyrate and whirl a cage with a bird on a green sponge an earthen deer a captive a strawberry fallen into cream a bonbonnière of dreams our muses do not resemble suburban heroines or a manhattan coconut from whose cavity springs a striped DANDY adept at hoax

small sailboat engine this hydra of our days is here that we may more easily pursue our chimeras brass hearts water nymphs drying their laundry on moonbeam clotheslines three kings chasing phantoms of the physical geography of cake ox-eye daisies

SHAFTS OF THE HEART

bored with everything we have conceived our repertoire from things we thus far consider innocent foremost CAMARGO ladies' shoes still life in seaweed the unfading calyxes of chandeliers among them eros disguised as a TRICKSTER tombs mills gloves roulette seascapes in a cabin of obscurities peonies of a divan under a child's exercise book lakes of cocktails

TRACKS OF MADNESS

strolling through the marketplaces of europe rid of the obligation to write letters to family we bought up each and every innocent young girl and prostitute so that by having nothing ADVENTURE would finally open to us

puppets, an atlas of polynesian butterflies of balloons a pony from a merry-go-round spitting out sugar cubes cabinets wonderment cummerbund

DREAM TAMER

we are harried by thoughts of artificial paradises ANYWHERE IN THE WORLD dutch windmills above the shanghai gates vacuous spaces nameless forms machinery of the hesperides orestes amid the furies ultimately PATHELIN[4] having on his robe the constellation of the Cross under whose sign pray poets no longer drinking white coffee

THE FAN OF SLEEP

artificial lunatics crawling along spiderwebs and superimposed on one another like the tone of a rattle shape overlays musicology form coinciding with the idea is a trap for analogy we catch with a butterfly net magical tea the sovereignty of crown paint colors but in the end it is white from the island of melos pale blue armenion and washed saudarah

LASTLY

the precursors of those who at the fin de siècle will flee from this century

Štyrský & Toyen
à votre service
Paris, 1926

[4] The husband and wife Pierre and Guilamette Pathelin are the main characters in the medieval French farce *La Farce de maître Pathelin*.

The Poet

(lecture delivered at an art opening)

Artificialism identifies the painter with the poet. This identification is indivisible, intrinsic, and simultaneous. It is not a fusion of painting and poetry, as such a fusion is non-simultaneous, extrinsic, and divisible. We couldn't care less about the label "Artificialism." We have used it only to differentiate and to separate this work from the excrement of so-called modern painting, to which we owe nothing.

We shall call the painter a poet.

Cubism took stock of traditional painting, divided into figurative, landscape, and still life. At root Cubism was a new a way to represent models with varying degrees of descriptiveness. It viewed the painting through the prism of a model. It replaced trompe l'oeil with the illusion of reality spatially disseminated and projected the illusion of space into reality. Forms in the painting coincided with forms in reality, and where this fragmentary casting proved impossible it gave way to distortion. This dissection bore fruit : duplication. Rather than activate the imagination, the Cubist painter skewed reality. Cubism achieved maximum reality. Then the wretch discovered it had no wings. It was betrayed by its own vision, with one eye squinting at reality and the other at the painting. This second eye has so failed to hold us in its thrall that we feel no visceral disgust at the quartering of the victim.

Constructivism and nonfigurative painting — nothing more than eye candy relying on a play of forms — resemble school writing exercises. Words precede thoughts, and people bear only the weight of words. As everything in the world has already been said and depicted, we need to build on effects, not causes. Primitive man, harried by fate and geometry, had a right to happiness. The poet is harried by chance. He resolves to eat a banana if it's been peeled. The Constructivists peeled Pythagoras, but ingested only his skin.

Artificialism rejects the trickery of figurative and literary historicism and distortion — this is Surrealism. The shorter our life the more fatuous similes we choose for it. We cannot haggle over terms, only over their ambit. The unconscious is a gag many stick in their mouths to keep from having to think. One generation bequeaths to the next a veneration for the sauce in which the world is stewed.

Rivers empty into cemeteries and the sea swallows ships in a never-ending quest for its swans. Swans with double necks, one that swallows sleep the other that regurgitates it. The magician devours applause in advance, forgetting he will not have the opportunity to puke it back up. Carrying wormwood, Noah's Ark founders. A mealworm sits on a branch and sings. The poet repudiates only its method.

Each one of us shadows our own toad, but its games of peekaboo elude human eyes. If we were to refind it, we could not be sure it's indeed our toad. Higher animals grow fat and the lower procreate. One day a hairy manikin will seize control of the world. Blue tunics will dig up graves and rob poets of their gold, then, having achieved equality, leave them in peace. Death will be nothing more than leaving the world of paper money. Gold will belong to the gravediggers, and the perfidious skies will swallow up doves and airplanes with equal benevolence. Only then will the airplanes start to sing.

Folks want only their daily soup, and manage to wait for it and take joy in it. Absurd theories are obligations we are free to interpret as we please without one having to yield to the other. The poet will untie the knot, throw away the key, and leave.

The dream bears out the experiences of our habits. We behold faces offensive with feigned bated breath. We cannot consider mendacious the weary smiles of flowers and collars. Many arrive and multiply the points of observation, swapping them until a chaos of the manifold emerges in the representation. Truth in the superfluous is the product of their snares. The mystery of their faces is on the outside, and time etches mendacity under their guise. We shall never know if the face has betrayed the likeness, if the likeness has deceived the actor, or if the face were simultaneously its own prompter and spectator. The only perfidy : to become convinced of your own mendacity.

The poet says goodbye to sleep. The hypocrite continues to pluck the names of flowers, but their true form does not exist. The thing's appearance would be embraced by a lyrical monster having as many eyes as the points in space encompassing the thing. The poet observes the appearance of things from the point of their origin.

The landscapes of dream are coulisses where the colors wait to fade, the light to be lit, and forms for the gigantic ruins to come. Life dispenses and returns expired pledges. Only the child is a spectator, chained to the grass and unable to leave if the performance turns terrifying. The secret of magicians is the pain they are able to bear, not that they don't feel any.

Having no microscopes, residents of the suburbs are not plagued by bedbugs. When drowning, we are irrevocably enticed by mirrors in which we might magnify our squalor. The poet is just now marching to the madhouse the Surrealists were driven out of long ago. You don't need to wander Oceania to find enchantment. The poet loves distances. Distances in time, not in space. The poet loves the earth at its beginning and at its end. A diluvial sea just inventing its language. No matter where the poet goes, he only needs the world he brings with him.

Poetry is not the continuation of the picture and the song prehistoric man began to compose. Mushrooms proliferate from a desire to imitate one another. Poetry arose from a desire to while away life.

In an era of celebrity, a rather thick layer of smegma has accumulated on the surreal, which cannot revive allusions to modern poets. The tattooing of the lower strata has seeped into the upper acting as counterpressure. The sham poet braces for his own depredation. Sleep reproduces the roots of his treachery. Cruel consciousness does not tinker with humility. The eyes gazing from the unconscious have heavy lids. Mirrors read from eyes. The victim weeps. He can no longer speak through sight. The gardener cultivates ribbons for future biers. Many contrive critical nitpicking. It was enough for the poet to observe how a nest is made by those who build on sleep while at the same time it is being ravished by those who build on the unconscious, yet he will not sit on the eggs with them. To build on the unconscious is to set store by deprivation.

Sleep is a bee hoarding honey so that a memory might savor it. We have no memories but are attempting to construct them. If this is the only way to be rid of memories. To have them leave us.

The poet employs colors or words to dilute what he wishes to say. He has no instinct for self-preservation, and yet he lives. The engineer dreams. He designs a new globe. The poet is no longer astonished by the face of night, boxes, and people. You will not find him in a scrum of gawpers. You will always find him in its center astride his victim. His victims are useless forms from which the colors found on the human scrapheap have slipped.

The adversity of epigones is comical. It simulates the joy of poets.

It is difficult for the sensible person to reach a state of joy from oneself alone. The poet begins at this border and continues in the opposite direction. His joy comes from paper, clouds, space, and ultimately emptiness. His joy has no model or template.

The poet does not work with reality. He is drawn to poetry, filling in the gaps between real forms, and to the void that reality emanates. He responds to the latent poetry of interior forms. He invents and creates their exterior. Imagination has lost interest in what is born and dies. It infers memories, memories of memories, untethered from mind and experience. Memory and recollection each in turn play the role of executioner.

The poet gives shape and color to eidetic emotion. His perceptions are transfigured at inception. Memories pass through consciousness without leaving either a mark or fading. Their formation is neither real nor artificial. It is natural. The poet will not find happiness in artificial paradises.

Reality and the image repel one another. An incantation lies between them : the word. It does not describe a theme. Theme and the painting are one. The title provides a directive for titillation, yet it leaves the viewer isolated and alone with the painting. Memory fabricates.

Štyrský & Toyen

On Artificialism

A few years ago, the French journal *L'Esprit nouveau* ran a survey that asked if the Louvre should be burned down. The question incited the entire global milieu of cultural snobs, and many artists, philosophers, art dealers, and others responded for or against the idea. Those who were in favor of burning down the Louvre, and they were by and large the very top poets and artists from around the world, often found themselves in a rather unenviable position. In one well-known incident, Tristan Tzara, the founder of Dada and one of the greatest contemporary poets, was assaulted at Café de la Rotonde by students of the School of Fine Arts in Paris.

In my opinion, the existence of the Louvre today, with its celebrated Mona Lisa's smile and ranks of moldy canvases, restored a hundred times over, depicting outmoded Madonnas, pastoral idylls, and all that allurement bereft of historical context, means little. If the Louvre ceased to exist it would truly be a major loss since we would no longer be able to behold those lovely English ladies staring starry-eyed at the nudes of Giorgione and Titian, but it would hardly be an irreplaceable loss as we live our adventures in front of canvases much more fascinating, intoxicated by the gaze that has escaped the lidded eyes of sultry Greta Garbo and Brigitte Helm. The faces of worldly beauties and chaste Renaissance Madonnas are so vapid, expressionless, entirely devoid of passion, that to us they seem like decaying junk and a tedious bore.

We love the canvas of the movie screen, those split-second smiles and kisses that seem to last for an eternity, enchantment on the white surface. We admire only a single old master, and that is Leonardo da Vinci, yet it is Leonardo the inventor, engineer, sorcerer, writer, and organizer of bacchanalias who so captivates us.

Searching for the antecedents of art is an exercise in futility. Art in general is what it is and not what it once was. Defining art from a historical perspective at the same time defines what art should not presently be. If the contemporary painter or sculptor creates forms that have already lived their lives and are therefore now dead, they are antithetical to the interests of modern society, which has not succumbed to antiquarian perversion and has no love for dirty, fusty relics. The modern artist is aware that nothing is more protean and relative than the idea of beauty.

Ancient Egyptians designed and carved their sphinxes, which for us have lost their mystery. They sculpted their history in granite and marble from a desire to have their chimerical lives last for eternity. Yet as we have come to know, only stone defies the centuries. The art of the ancient Egyptians is dead to us, and their stories hold little interest. If Egypt does happen to beguile our imagination, then it is not the Egypt of the pharaohs but the banks of the eternally blue Nile, the oases on the edge of the desert. Our age has more lofty pursuits than the excavation of pharaohs or the draining of Lake Nemi, which ate up millions to uncover several rotted beams to the disintegrating frame of a common boat such as the hundreds anchored in the coal harbor of Genoa.

Whoever admires ancient art will never create a new art, an art for today. The modern painter only learns how not to paint from old masters and at the Academy. But he's never told how he should paint. At one time, and it wasn't that long ago, it was thought that the modern artist would benefit more by learning from house painters and varnishers. Though this might sound like utter nonsense, without this sort of training Fernand Léger, for one, is unthinkable. He learned by observing the multicolored motley of posters plastered on the street corner.

The modern painter learns everywhere, though his work does not accord with nature or models. Nature and the world have become patterns, an inventory of forms, shapes, colors, nuances from which he amalgamates his paradise. One day he spots the subtleties of a pink cloud floating westward, and transforms this hue in his mind into the velvety neck of a girl he once kissed. With these feelings recalled, he creates, and his work evokes in the perceptive viewer a sense of tenderness long lost and rediscovered. Viewers then mechanically reify this sensation for themselves.

People today are laborers. They are worn out. They need a non-destructive art, they need enchantment, they need poetry. The age of spleen, coffee klatches, dark vigils, and the dankness of the family hearth has long passed. It was an age that directly engendered Nietzsche, Wagner, and Munch, to name only a few, and they were persons who needed art to expend themselves and to galvanize their degenerate indolence. To be sure, I am not speaking here in favor of facile muses, or in favor of kitsch, folk, and proletarian art. I would only like to emphasize that art needs to be divested of meditation, symbol, bias, and didacticism. This does not give, however, the snobs, dilettantes, and retrograde painters the right to disparage the modern painter as a trendy, shallow acrobat.

The modern work of art can only be appreciated by someone who is vital, someone whose intellectual pursuits and incessant, onerous flux of life have not been engulfed by the mass of affections welling up from the unconscious. Those who disparage the modern painter only prove how malnourished they are.

Until recently, there was much talk about painting and photography competing with one another, and yet it is abundantly clear no such competition exists. Photography shows us objective events and a slice of time that is a factual record, a faithful reproduction, exact. There is not a more veracious witness, and nothing has the ability to inform as precisely as the photograph. For this reason, photography has been closely associated with journalism and reportage. It has the feel of the real world in which we live. It is one-hundred percent reality in all its optical and spatial truth.

While Illusionism has no place in painting, it is a virtue in photography and constitutes its pure realism. An example of good realism in photography, that is, objective, dispassionate photographs, perfectly simulates reality. An example of the bad, that is, nonobjective photography, simulates printmaking, such as that done by František Drtikol[5] in Prague.

The evolution of photography and film, however, expedited the evolution of the fine arts. The dreams of the old masters have been realized, because their ideal as painters was imitation, and they indirectly indicated the paths painting should shun. When Ingres painted his renowned *The Turkish Bath,* he knew nothing of photography. This painting grabs us because the artist was attempting to objectively depict reality as he saw it. If we envisage a Turkish bath today in film, clearly we can no longer paint it à la Ingres, or depict things like in the photograph. Since the Neoclassicists and Neorealists

5 Czech photographer (1883–1961) famous for his nudes, portraits, and experimental photography.

failed to understand this, their work is full of egregious errors. Take our own Otakar Kubín[6] in Paris. It is not the modern painting's function to be narrative, epic, or genre. Even so, it still retains its dramatic quality. The painter converts the old literary dramatic quality inherent in the subject matter into the drama of forms, colors, and space. The painting has become purely a lyrical world unto itself. The first to comprehend this were the Cubists Picasso and Braque.

The process of creating a photograph is purely mechanical. The process of creating a painting is at heart the creation of a new reality. As soon as modern painting found itself in this realm, it discovered new and unlimited poetic possibilities.

I would like to return for a moment to the past, even though to my mind when this world contains both the old and the new it makes more sense to dwell on the latter, or at least on things not too distant in the past. I'll skip those perennial images of the Crucifixion and the Madonna, immersed in funereal black and faded brown, and pass over the Classicists, French naturalism, and stop at the Impressionists. Like you, I, too, was in thrall in my youth to these tremors of light. Recall Monet's gardens and Renoir's young girls. Recall Seurat, who took the theory of Impressionism to its logical conclusion and who is considered the first precursor of modern painting. After him came that angry father Cézanne, whose paintings were a working out of equations and are still interesting today only for those who continue to conceive painting as a multiplication table. Contemporary painting is too distant from these pursuits to return to the galleries and museums. Lastly, Le Douanier Rousseau — the painting seen through the eyes of a child and executed by an artless hand with the thick fingers of a dilettante.

Rousseau is simply an anachronism in painting even with his ponies, brides, and the springtime Seine. There is such a concentration of popular poetic sentiment in Rousseau that if he had been born a painter rather than a dilettante he would've been a great painter. His Primitivism is completely alien to the present, and his work is entirely hermetic, because the modern person is looking for greater sophistication, not trite primitivism, to offset the fatigue from mechanical contemporary life. In his life

[6] Czech painter (1883–1969) associated with Post-Impressionism, Kubín became a French citizen in 1925 and went by the name Othon Coubine.

and work the Czech painter Jan Zrzavý[7] resembles Rousseau. The others — Matisse, Derain, Kisling, Utrillo, Dufy, Laurencin, Modigliani, et al. — fill in the gaps. Their work sells, they are celebrated, but the future will remember little more than their names and a few of their artworks. Modern painting begins anew with Picasso and Braque.

Cubism evolved over twenty years, and only recently has developed further by branching out into several directions. Cubism was in fact less exceptional than is commonly held. The Cubist painter unpacked the shapes of individual things to represent them more vividly and completely. He arranged shapes in relation to one another in the picture to create space while giving the composition balance. Because it placed the greatest emphasis on the picture plane, Cubism at first distorted objects, but later, when it had switched back toward objectivity, it distorted space and fastidiously refrained from balancing out the picture plane. This was the period when Picasso was pasting scraps of newspaper, wood, matches, hair, glass, etc. onto the surface of the painting. Braque abandoned Cubism in the years immediately after the war, while Picasso was just beginning to draw on his many years of experimenting : his paintings had a surface balance that did not display his previous errors to such a degree that they would bury him or cause him to give up his efforts. His imitators proliferated : Albert Gleizes, Juan Gris, Léopold Survage, and others, such as our own Emil Filla.[8]

Even though modern painting is unthinkable without Cubism, it did nothing more than synthesize the outcomes of traditional painting, which was categorized as figurative, landscape, and still life with varying degrees of descriptiveness. At root Cubism was merely a new way to represent objects. It replaced trompe l'oeil with the illusion of reality spatially disseminated. It generally viewed the painting through the prism of a model. Pictorial forms either coincided with real forms, or where this proved impossible, they gave way to distortion. The Cubist painter dissected the world in a way that

7 Painter, graphic artist, and illustrator, Jan Zrzavý (1890–1977) was an important early modernist Czech artist associated with Symbolism.

8 An early adopter of Cubism, Filla (1882–1953) was one of the leading Czech avant-garde artists of the prewar period.

was more scientific than intuitive, thus all it achieved was a mirroring, a duplication. Where the Cubist painter erred, therefore, was in skewing reality rather than activating his own imagination. When Picasso had achieved the maximum illusion of reality he began to have eyes for the origins of Cubism, and through German Expressionism and French Classicism came back to African sculpture. Cubism's offshoot, the Purism of Ozenfant and Jeanneret (Le Corbusier), did nothing more than apply to painting the catchwords of Purism in architecture, and today it has already been abandoned by its creators.

Italian Futurism, which emerged during the same period as Cubism, attempted to capture the movement of things in space. When Boccioni exhibited his first mosaic paintings in 1913, Picasso had already created some important works of art. With the gradual evolution of film, which captures movement directly, Futurism fell into decline as an anachronism, an already dated artistic form. Boccioni and Severini died[9] and their confrère Carrà began to produce kitsch.

Mondrian's Neoplasticism, or painting without a representational function, creating pure relationships between lines and color, was a reaction to the decline of Cubism and the first real step toward total abstraction in painting.

Before looking at modern painting, Surrealism and Artificialism, I would first like to say a few words about how seven years ago we were searching for new directions away from Cubism.

We began with the premise that the picture is the poetry of sight, a poetic vision of the world. Such a vision can never be realistic even though it is born out of reality and from real elements. It has no consistent space and no consistent pattern. It is neither window nor display case. It is above all a surface, despite all its concrete elements. Out of a need to augment this surface with the magic of words, we inscribed or drew on the picture various slogans, sentences, etc., which became part of the image. True, the Cubists also had done this, but the difference was that their words were only meant to be decorative and communicated nothing to the viewer.

This was how the picture poem emerged without the image being reduced to the

[9] Severini actually died in 1966.

level of illustration. We later replaced painted sections with photographs and discovered the photomontage when it was nothing more than a dream in Russia. So we manipulated reality in photomontages and in paintings, not as a method of representation or of breaking down reality purely for the purposes of representation, but to express its innate poetry. The picture thus became a kaleidoscope that had no need of logic, the same as beauty has no need of logic. Pictorial, spatial, and perspective issues no longer needed to be addressed as these pictures were predominantly lyrical, yet a lyricism that was not an end in itself like with the abstract arabesques found in Kupka's Orphism or Malevich's Surprematism.

We discussed materials at length. We studied the chemical makeup of pigments, optics, and the physiological effect of color, line, and surface. We considered the suitability of oil paint as a modern material in the hands of the artist. We combined the techniques of painting with other materials, taking as inspiration Apollinaire's words that a good painter could use any material to paint with, such as with blood during the French Revolution or with feces.[10] Thus our schooling was more complex and more scientific than any art academy could ever have provided.

We devoted much attention to learning the techniques of reproduction because it was our dream to print our pictures according to our own specifications while being careful not to get bogged down in handcraft.

I don't know why, but the public became inured to our work and called what we produced Constructivism. This is still a mystery to us because save for Karel Teige not one of us has ever had anything in common with the Constructivists, who have flooded the stage, the pages of books, and so forth with their formulaic designs.

Now I will try to say a few words about Surrealism, or Surrealist painting. Surrealism is a direct outgrowth of Dada, and though it has made some contributions to literature, it's made a more indelible mark in painting. Surrealism is defined as pure psychic automatism in order to express the actual functioning of thought.[11] Surrealism subordinates thought, poetry, painting, etc. to chance as it is based on a faith in higher

10 See Guillaume Apollinaire, *Les Peintres Cubistes, Méditations Esthétiques* (Paris, 1913).

11 See André Breton, "Manifesto of Surrealism" (1924).

forms of association that have thus far been ignored, a faith in the omnipotence of dream and in the play of the mind as an end in itself. The Surrealist mode of creation is based on the subconscious dictate of thought entirely outside the control of reason, entirely outside any consideration of aesthetics and morality.

Drawing on Freud, the Surrealists hold that the dream is an expression of our essential being. Like their colleagues of a literary bent, Surrealist painters have chronicled their dreams and in so doing have created a type of absurd oneiric reality. They record lines, surfaces, and marks without any sort of rational organization or regard to what the outcome might be. As a result, these surrealistic paintings, for which no aesthetic criteria of modern painting can be applied nor any standard imposed [. . .][12] resemble mediumistic drawings and the works of madmen in a state the French call *fous discordants*. They are lunatics whose memories and fantasies are preserved in their consciousness but whose visual associations are diffused in other collapsed mental realities. The surrealistic painting often gives the impression of being illustration, or of having an odious literary taint, which is further bolstered by the painter's poor technical skill and, more often than not, utter incompetence, even though the painting itself is conceived rather poetically. Chirico is the sole exception. But he was already a good painter prior to Surrealism. The Surrealist painters worth mentioning are : Francis Picabia, Joan Miró, André Masson, Paul Klee, Yves Tanguy, and Josef Šíma.

To conclude I would like to talk about my paintings and Toyen's paintings and Artificialism.

Artificialism identifies the painter with the poet. The modern painter must likewise be a poet. This identification is indivisible, intrinsic, and simultaneous, therefore Artificialism is not a fusion of painting and poetry, as it was with the so-called picture poem, where the fusion was non-simultaneous, where each component could exist independently of the other. We couldn't care less about the label Artificialism. We have used it only to differentiate and to separate this work from the whole of so-called modern painting.

Striving for a maximum of imagination, we do not work with reality. We reject

12 Lacuna in original.

painting as merely a play of form and eye candy. We do not deny the existence in a painting of real elements divested of their objectiveness, but we do not work with them. Our sole focus is poetry, which fills the gap between real forms, poetry, which reality emanates. A poetry of interiority.

The function of the intellect is extrinsic and finite. It organizes and disciplines and to an extent burnishes the emotional payoff.

The Artificialist painting is not bound to reality under conditions of time, locus, and space, therefore it does not lend itself to any associative visions.

Artificialism arises from each color being subjected on its own to the effects of light, thus any anomaly of diffuse and condensed light produces no changes in it. Lyrical ambience is created by color value and transposition.

The composition of a painting, having arisen from a disinterest in reality, assumes total awareness and is contingent on the concrete logic of the Artficialist painting. Forms in the painting coincide with eidetic memory. The title given the painting, therefore, is neither caption nor thematic appellation, but is indicative of its emotive character. Theme and the painting are one. Its forms are self-explanatory. The merit of Artificialism will be in allowing the modern painter to be called a poet.

A poet.

Each one of us shadows our own toad, but its games of peekaboo elude human eyes. If we were to refind it, we could not be sure it's indeed our toad. Higher animals grow fat and the lower procreate. One day a hairy manikin will seize control of the world. Blue tunics will dig up graves and rob poets of their gold, then, having achieved equality, leave them in peace. Death will be nothing more than leaving the world of paper money. Gold will belong to the gravediggers, and the perfidious skies will swallow up doves and airplanes with equal benevolence. Only then will the airplane start to sing.

The poet says goodbye to sleep. The hypocrite continues to pluck the names of flowers, but their true form does not exist. The thing's appearance would be embraced by a lyrical monster having as many eyes as the points in space encompassing the thing. The poet observes the appearance of things from the point of their origin.

You don't need to wander Oceania to find enchantment. The poet loves distances. Yet distances in time, not in space. The poet loves the earth at its beginning and at its end. A diluvial sea just inventing its language. No matter where the poet goes, he only needs the world he brings with him.

Poetry is not the continuation of the pictures and the song prehistoric man began to compose. Mushrooms proliferate from a desire to imitate one another. Poetry arose from a desire to while away life.

The poet employs colors and words to dilute what he wishes to say. He has no instinct for self-preservation, and yet he lives. The engineer dreams. He designs a new globe.

It is difficult for the sensible person to reach a state of joy from oneself alone. The poet begins at this border and continues in the opposite direction. His joy come from paper, clouds, and ultimately emptiness. His joy has no model or template.

The poet always leaves the viewer isolated and alone.

A Generation's Corner

I

Our generation has come of age : it identifies the moon with the electric bulb, love with the bed, poetry with the purse. It measures quality by the level of success and conquers life by brown-nosing. Many have grown old and shabby, and time has changed the imperceptible, microscopic signs of mental poverty into the massive ulcer of mental destitution. Others satisfied their cravenness. They so elevated their wretchedness as to be considered two-bit layabouts with impunity. Comfortably ensconced in seclusion, they're enjoying their thirty pieces of silver. The absurdity of their lives is rooted in the fact that their actual merit has never attained the level of their reputation. Every so often they mirror the appearance of movement, like bulrushes reflected on a pond surface. They secretly malign one another without any loss of self-respect. Although they have an extremely idyllic view of the world, they form an aggregate much more complex than might be assumed, since the more mercenary they are, the less firm their grasp of kitsch, or better put, the more self-indulgent they are, the more kitsch they produce. Their acumen is excellent. It is a generation that dreams of bathtubs. *The only place today for the true poet is the pillory.*

Our generation likes to blather about adventure and the outré, while in truth there's never been a more docile herd. It has presumed to gird the whole world yet never managed to determine its own capacity. This generation's trajectory from the outset was linked to the annihilation of others' joy, in which it reveled. With each attempt to widen their horizons a lamb was sacrificed. The nation has already erected monuments to many of them. Portrayed seated, a patina covers their youth.

Surely it is more rewarding to love illusions, since they are impenetrable, than to believe in them, since we live in them. It seems we are going to disdain for a long time to come the youth *of others,* who will wend their way among coteries coming and going, quietly *retrogressing* in the midst of universal development and progress to maintain life's eternal equilibrium. Each generation has to be driven out by whatever weapon it most deserves. Rather than the butcher's cleaver or the rapier, it seems the most appropriate for our generation is a dash of strychnine.

People of today, or their symbol, their trace, have lapsed into error, for they would like to be convinced by *smell* of the fragility of a rose, whose image is hidden in their unconscious, which is in such constant flux that no *eye* can follow it and makes it impossible to form any plausible idea of a rose. It will always be just a rose, evoking horror. Even if a single machine were to perform the work of hundreds of thousands of human hands in the future, humans would still demolish it purely from these hands having nothing better to do.

Poetry's future does not lie in the cleverness a generation advances. No generation has had more printed pages, more incense, parasites, clowns, narcissists, good fortune, and Elberfeld horses than ours, and yet no generation has had fewer poets. It has paid dearly for its cleverness. Every moron born at a certain time claims membership.

It is time to put an end to the myth of a generation so that the imbeciles who've comfortably and serenely set up shop in it might after a confetti moment also enjoy the pleasures of the mind, that is, their *invisibility*. And so that those who've prostituted themselves might blush one last time.

Sitting on two chairs is as brazen as harboring the secret wish to lie in two graves.

Our generation is disintegrating. A few poets still live the way they want. For them the earth rests heavily and the distance lightly.[13] Or vice versa.

II

I was taken to task for the fact that the first part of "A Generation's Corner" created such a furor, though not an entirely honest furor. Yet I fear it might be misused in the places where I would least expect it. Naturally, I didn't react to the commentary of certain circles to my article, as these comments were directed more at a generation's particular corner than at me, and they brought me no joy, no grief, and no diarrhea.

I am not looking for the meaning of life here so as to play judge or hangman of a generation. It's not something to which my physical constitution or abilities are suited,

13 An allusion to the Latin funerary inscription: *Sit tibi terra levis.*

so I'll leave this honorable function to those jaded folk who don't faint in the presence of the most bizarre individuals parading around in their underclothes. I've encapsulated my opinion in a pill, and while perhaps "addling" at first, I do not intend despite this presumed downside to dilute it in water.

I find my article completely without ambiguity, and I consider my words definitive. I hope each is able to see it for what it is.

I would only like to make a few remarks : I was amused to no end to learn that many took my statement, *"The only place today for the true poet is the pillory,"* to mean a stake of some sort, chained to which is a Villonesque vagabond, looking like one of those loudmouths from political meetings and holding in his hand (calloused naturally) the insignia of a particular party.

I am amazed that Karel Teige used my article, directly citing several lines from it, to support his own arguments in the Vančura affair, which, let it be said once and for all, is nobody's business.[14]

My article had no political subtext. I was talking primarily about the purity of the work, about literary prostitution, and it should be clear from my words that *for me the modern poet is someone who has not betrayed his work.* I think it's clear as day that my words "so that those who've prostituted themselves might blush one last time" have been taken out of context by Teige. He would have been better served if he had written about Vančura in connection with his own words at the end of his article : *"Fortunately there is something more solid than any 'generation' : fidelity to one's work, opinion, orientation, a belief in international community."* It's such a shame that Teige does not employ his leadership abilities and combative élan more in matters of poetry and that his interest in politics has lately taken precedence over his interest in poetry.

I consider the total conflation of those spirits of revolution with the revolutionary spirits in art fatuous and a residue of a reactionary attitude in the worlds of both

[14] In 1929, Vladislav Vančura and six other writers quit the Communist Party of Czechoslovakia in protest to its Bolshevization under the new leadership headed by Klement Gottwald. In addition to using Štyrský's text to call for a purge, Teige attacked Vančura for having accepted the State Prize for Literature. And he then responded to "A Generation's Corner (II)" by calling it "the most idiotic article ever written in our country against revolutionary avant-garde artists."

politics and art. It is a negative of patriotic paradises. It makes little difference if the poet is a paperboy for *Rudé právo*[15] or a general in the Czechoslovak Army, as difficult as this might be to imagine. The true poet always stands apart from political machinations and demagoguery. Revolution always appropriates the poet only ex post.

Of course, I wouldn't want to make this a generally applicable rule, even though history, past and present, has generally shown that the most progressive revolutionaries, politicians, sociologists, state economists who play such important roles in contemporary life were on the whole the greatest reactionaries when it came to art. And it should also be said that the poet is on the whole completely indifferent to political coups or radical social changes or class upheavals. Whoever is familiar with Baudelaire knows that his revolutionary activity in 1848 was an entirely minor episode in his life and that he was not a poet of the Revolution. Nor was J. A. Rimbaud, who joined the Commune for the very banal reason that he was hungry. He was not a Communard for even a month before he fled Paris in advance of that legendary bloody week. I could likewise name Jules Laforgue, Nerval, Germaine Nouveau, Lautréamont, Mallarmé, and Apollinaire.

A poet's interests always lie outside political parties — he doesn't lollygag with a tricolored patriotic pin in his lapel and couldn't care less how much 50 grams of cinnamon cost in the USSR.

The poet has rid himself of all bias. He admires the heroes of the Revolution the same as the heroes of the counterrevolution. If he should love death, then the execution of Sacco and Vanzetti excites him in the same way as the execution of the tsar's family. Etc.

The poet is berated as egocentric and antisocial, while from the *right and left* hyenas howl at both his deeds and his verse. Both the good and bad of human society are the poet's enemy.

Yes : *The pillory is the only place the true poet belongs.*

[15] *Rudé právo* [Red Justice] was founded in 1920 as the official newspaper of the Communist Party of Czechoslovakia.

III

In *Odeon,*[16] no. 3, I published an article that was taken by a certain group of leftist cultural operatives as a backflip, with some ascribing to it a retrograde political tendency. And one fine fellow (Karel Teige) even reared his head to use my piece as a pretext for emptying his bladder of the personal bile filling it (see *Tvorba,* nos. 23 and 24[17]). I think it's ludicrous and unnecessary to polemicize with these types of articles. I can only express regret at Teige's behavior, which lately has verged on the ridiculous. In *Tvorba,* no. 24, I published a few remarks pertaining to my article in the last issue of *Odeon*. It can be taken as my response to Julius Fučík, Ivan Sekanina, and Ladislav Štoll.[18]

Both of Teige's texts in *Tvorba* show his chaotic thought process, though to be sure he is less concerned with ideas and matters of principle than with the "case of Jindřich Štyrský."

I have nothing personal against Teige. I concede his undeniable service to modern Czechoslovak culture, even though clearly *his activity has never been creative.* He has always been a compiler, and the whole of his work is nothing but a compilation of others' knowledge, others' theories, others' artistic approaches, others' work, etc.

Once the torchbearer in a wasteland, today Teige senses his own superfluousness. He has nothing new to offer. And this is the source of his hysteria and his arrant spinsterhood. Teige's greatness lay in his ability to quickly assimilate the ideas and outcomes of others' work and to take this paradoxical and complex bonanza that had come his way and toss fistfuls of it all around him until nothing was left for himself.

16 The magazine *Odeon – Literární kurýr* [Literary Courier Odeon] was published from 1929 to 1931 by Jan Fromek and edited by Jindřich Štyrský.

17 A biweekly leftist magazine for "literary, political, and art criticism" founded in 1925 by the leading literary critic F.X. Šalda and literary historian Otokar Fischer.

18 Julius Fučík (1903–43) was a hack and prominent member of the Czechoslovak Communist Party, writing both for *Rudé právo* and *Tvorba*. Active in the anti-Nazi resistance, he was imprisoned, tortured, and hanged in Germany. Ivan Sekanina (1900–40) was a left-wing journalist and lawyer on the payroll of the Communist Party. An anti-fascist activist, he was arrested soon after Nazi Germany occupied the Czech lands in March 1939 and ultimately died in Sachsenhausen. Ladislav Štoll (1902–81) was a Marxist literary critic, editor of *Rudé právo* from 1934, and prominent postwar Communist politician and MP in the National Assembly.

I see in this his personal tragedy and failure. The Teige case could be demonstrated by what I wrote in *Odeon,* no. 1, about a generation that blathers about adventure and the outré while in truth it belongs to the most docile herd. It presumes to gird the whole world while never managing to determine its own capacity, and its trajectory is linked to the annihilation of others' joy, in which it revels. — The absurdity of their lives is rooted in the fact that their actual merit has never attained the level of their reputation.

Karel Teige is not exactly the complicated person his writings would like us to believe. From the beginning his work has been merely a denial of himself, and this is why today Teige is nothing other than his own miscarried caricature. *Look at all that K. Teige aspired to be :* poet, writer, journalist, filmmaker, painter, caricaturist, literary and art critic, architect, editor, music and film aesthetician, typographer, commercial artist, etc. etc. *And look at what K. Teige is today.*

His literary and artistic output has been a series of absurd contradictions. Teige proclaimed the renaissance of realistic primitivism, he proclaimed collective folk art, and then immediately pursued Cubism and wrote a monograph on Jan Zrzavý. In a fit of disgust with everything, he later declared the liquidation of art while gripping the coattails of Ilya Ehrenburg. During this period he began to produce photomontages à la Rodchenko, calling them picture poems, and authored the Manifesto of Poetism, all the while engaged in a feeble flirtation with Dada and declaring the primacy of Constructivism. Etc., etc.

I have sketched this portrait of our little jack-of-all-trades without getting personal and with quite a bit of regret, considering his better past.

Teige has called me "an unproductive painter for some time now." I would reproach myself for being discourteous to him if I had neglected to invite him to my exhibition (February 1930 at the Aventinum). I hope he will like my work, as he has up till now. Of course, my exhibition runs the risk that he'll then feel compelled to say that I've been an unproductive writer for some time now.

When I wrote the first part of "A Generation's Corner," Teige viciously chastised me for not naming names, for not pointing a finger at these individuals, and today

I suppose he would chastise me again that I've only singled him out.

The next issue of *Odeon* will contain a number of articles *purely on foundational ideas and principles,* and future issues will no longer address the problems and fortunes of particular individuals, leaving such personal squabbles to the weeklies, such as *Tvorba,* which has, so it seems, given them a permanent place in its pages.

I am not, nor have I ever been . . .

I am not, nor have I ever been, involved in a Communist organization, and neither is anyone I am associated with, such as Nezval, Teige, et al. I have never taken part in a labor movement nor in the Communist Party — nor, it goes without saying, in any other party. This was and is known about me. Julius Fučík certainly knew this when in *Tvorba,* no. 13, he ran my article "A Generation on Two Chairs."[19] *My attitude toward Communism was and is positive.*

I am astonished that my text in *Odeon,* no. 3, has been taken as a betrayal and an attempt to side with the reactionary camp. As a whole, the text was attacking trash and kitsch regardless where it's found, on the Right or on the Left. So naturally those who shield trash and kitsch would take umbrage at it. In this regard I am compelled to name Karel Teige.

I maintain that the total conflation of the revolutionary spirits in politics with the revolutionary spirits in art is utter nonsense. Besides, this was explained by Ivan Sekanina in *Tvorba,* no. 22, where he pointed out that such a conflation brings no benefit to either the Revolution or poetry.

My statement that revolution appropriates poets was poorly formulated (given how it was interpreted). What I meant was that poets are appropriated by revolutionary critics of the type and character represented by Karel Teige.

I did not mean to say that the poet has no interest in social issues or political questions, but that the poet is most certainly not an *activist.* For example, I am a member of the Left Front[20] because the whole orientation of my current work belongs there and because this association does not dictate to me that I play an *active* political role.

19 A reprint of "A Generation's Corner" with commentary from Julius Fučík.

20 The *Levá fronta* was established in December 1929 as an organization of avant-garde leftist artists associated with the Communist Party of Czechoslovakia, even though it formally claimed no political affiliations.

When I wrote that the true poet always keeps his distance from political machinations and demagoguery, then I think I was telling the truth, and naturally I think it right to suppose that revolutions and liberation movements are something more than mere political machination. The words I penned about loudmouths at political meetings should have been more precise by stating that these loudmouths are those who use their political influence and convictions only when something is to be gained by it and are silent when it comes to a friend.

I do not intend to let myself be shoved by anyone into the corner where many from this generation already find themselves or are taking the best route to reach while Karel Teige remains completely silent (which is why I chide him the most).

The Drawings of Writers

The forays of writers into the visual arts oftentimes bring more enjoyment than the so-called immortal creations in museums. The drawings of writers do not differ in any fundamental way from what is commonly produced by dilettantes, except that what we call subject matter in the drawings of dilettantes here we could call a motif. And though this classification might seem paradoxical, as writers normally limn real imagery and concrete facts and refrain from expressing any emotional state, which is what most dilettantes do via symbols either directly or indirectly, such drawings have very little to do with the creative process. Always conscious of the inferiority of their work, the writer who draws hurdles a thousand coincidences and forswears the many trivialities to which the common dilettante, thinking his work important, often succumbs. The writer who draws resembles a child at play, while the dilettante who draws most often resembles a card sharp, and as such traffics in fraud, hypocrisy, and admiration for the game of skill. Thus the efforts of the dilettante often end in virtuosity, conventional artistry, bombast.

Drawings by writers, however, show a lack of general technical skill and formal definition, save a few exceptions, such as the concrete poetry of Jean Cocteau, and therefore they have meaning and importance as a subject only for literary historians and lovers of curiosities. It would be a mistake to try to glean anything of relevance in the drawings of writers and poets to gain deeper insight into their work. The poet is playing. Relaxing. He only continues to draw by force of habit, triggering a recollection of life before he learned to read and write.

The earliest writer we know of who also dabbled in the visual arts is Euripides. After him history records a long list of names of famous writers and poets whose graphic art has come down to us. These include : Petrarch, Voltaire, Goethe, Nikolaus Lenau, Victor Hugo, Daudet, Théophile Gautier, Heinrich Heine, Prosper Mérimée, Baudelaire, Dostoevsky, Alfred de Musset, Verlaine, Rimbaud, Jules Laforgue, Karel Hlaváček, Jehan Rictus, Hugues Rebell, Charles Fort, E.T.A. Hoffmann, Barbey d'Aurevilly, K.H. Mácha, Anatol France, Pierre Loti, Robert Louis Stevenson, Gabriele D'Annunzio, the Goncourts, Alfred Jarry, Charles Péguy, Remy de Gourmont, Arthur Symons, Jean Moréas, Francis Carco, Paul Valéry, Max Jacob, Mac Orlan, Paul Morand, Jean Cocteau, Tristan Tzara, etc. etc.

There are many anecdotes on how these drawings came into being. Georges Hugo relates how his grandfather, Victor Hugo, would have a printer's sheet of paper brought to him after lunch, and on it he would proceed to make random blots, some of which were then expanded into his more well-known drawings, depicting nocturnal landscapes, spooky castles, and romantic princesses.

Théophile Gautier drew and painted scenes from the tabloids, balls, and carnivals of the day long before he devoted himself to literature. His favorite subject was Egyptian Nile landscapes. But even later, at the height of his fame as a writer, he continued to draw and paint, and his imaginary portrait of Mademoiselle de Maupin is unforgettable for its beauty. Émile Bergerat was right in saying about Gautier that his painter's palette did not have a thousandth part of the color of his writer's palette.

Verlaine's drawings are fairly well known, as is his morbid desire for pencil and paper that at times verged on a mania. He drew on scraps of paper, on magazines in cafés while drinking absinthe, he drew in the hospital on medical forms, and very few of his letters were not adorned with drawings.

The drawings of Baudelaire, which have a kind of equivalent in C. Guys,[21] are the best known to the public at large. He enjoyed drawing his own portrait, a face wracked with haphazard lines and absurd grimaces. Apollinaire's drawings are also widely known. Even as a child he drew strange images, very similar to the work of some Surrealist painters. His novella *The Poet Assassinated* was published in Paris and illustrated with his own gouaches. The examples of Jean Cocteau and Max Jacob would require their own studies.

Look at the nearly forgotten drawings of Alfred de Musset from his journey to Italy with George Sand. Gabriel Faure was the first in France to draw attention to

21 Constantin Guys (1802–92), Dutch-born correspondent during the Crimean War, illustrator for French and British newspapers, whom Baudelaire called the "painter of modern life."

them, having obtained permission for their publication from Musset's niece, Mme. Lardin de Musset.

Musset was clearly a talented draftsman. As a boy he copied some of the works in the Louvre of Italian masters, whose biographies he knew (he would later put this knowledge to use in his writings : *Andrea del Sarto* and *Le Fils du Titien*). In May 1833, he met Sand at a dinner party given by François Buloz for the editors of *Revue des deux Mondes,* and together they traveled to Italy in December of that same year. They took a diligence from Paris to Lyon and then to Avignon by boat. And on deck they met Stendhal, who was on his way to Civitavecchia to take up his position as the newly appointed consul. All three disembarked at Pont-Saint-Esprit and dined in one of the inns. In her memoirs, Sand writes that Stendhal got drunk and danced around the table in his high leather boots. — By all accounts the lovers were happy to part with their companion in Marseille, who continued overland to Italy. Musset and Sand left by ship. In the album there is another drawing depicting Musset suffering a painful bout of seasickness on the ship while Sand smokes a cigarette. After arriving in Genoa, the lovers continued on their way to Pisa. Musset drew Sand here holding a fan in a manner reminiscent of one of Gozzoli's beauties.

We know what happened next. Venice. Doctor Pagello. Sand's infidelity while Musset was bedridden with fever. During their stay, Musset did not draw and wrote only one thirteen-verse song : "A Saint-Blaise, à la Zuecca . . ." At the end of March 1834 a ravaged Musset left to return to France. Sand and Pagello accompanied him as far as Vicenza. He was alone. By April 10 he was back in Paris. He took solace in the arms of Aurore Dudevant. Sometimes he would peruse the album of his Italian trip. The silk covering the boards was becoming worn. These were Musset's last drawings.

On the Štyrský & Toyen Exhibition

We have separated ghastly gravestones from common cobblestones, we have stuck letters on the ledges of cottages, we have waited for the lethal blue of the sky, nearly lake blue. We think of a scroll of parchment resembling a candle in form and autumn in color when among hundreds of thousands of leaves a single maple leaf, inscribed with Talmudic tales, falls in the lane called Under the Bladdernut. Better to dress in sackcloth for this summer.

Thankfully, we never got bogged down in iconoclasm. We did not dress tree trunks in ladies gowns, nor did we assemble a celestial lesbian from trumpet and violin. We have debased imagination, as it may gratify anyone. We have arrived at places and regions more portentous than Lake Gérardmer or the Faust House and the hollow eyes of succubi, more than the legerdemain transposing realities into space, forms into abstractions, and vice versa. All those landscapes arising from tabletops, hundred headed women, and mannequins with breasts striated with the twigs of some mystical shrub are for us matters more peripheral than summer pads, factories, seaside resorts, morning stars, and female buttocks are for others.

While Surrealism has yet to create a "Cinderella" from poetry and a *Decameron* from painting, while it compromisingly teeters between the reproductive impulse and creating from dreams, between generating concepts of disequilibrium and the current penchant for comical subconscious superfluities, the last residues of a delirious Romanticism that has resulted in the symbol as analogy of the concrete and link to unconscious memory, while over this spectacle a flock of potatoes traverses the sky instead of clouds, we've stopped having illusions about things that are and are not beautiful : Pascal's brain, the locks of Lucrezia Borgia, a piece of smoked salmon, thoughts of suicide. We have tried to understand the difference between the method by which the typical schizophrenic preserves memories and the method by which the amateur photographer immortalizes a trip. Real life is not devoid of monstrosity. From this perspective, many things that generally seem to be complicated are revealed under an idiot's lamplight : for the melancholic, the blazing red of a flower is superfluous — the melancholic does not perceive even primary colors and sees everything in monochrome, most often in blue or ash-gray.

To see implies, in vulgar terms, to identify with the object.

When Leeuwenhoek in the 17th century first saw through his primitive microscope a realm of microbes in a drop of drinking water, his reaction was likely shock rather than joy. From this moment he looked at everything in a different light from others. The contents of a gob of spit immediately held for him greater value — if we can speak of it as *spectacle* — than the panorama spread out before his windows, on which the geraniums were in bloom.

To see also somewhat implies *blindness,* as there exist *landscapes of the visible and the invisible.*

Recent Books

Vítězslav Nezval, *Strach* [Fear], Drama, Edice Pražské Saturnalie, Prague, 1930

After the deluge of J. Cocteau's poeticized stage banalities, V. Nezval has spurned the so-called modern devices of the modern theater. He wrote this play without feeling the need either to magnify human fates or examine human passions under a microscope. Instead of a person, Nezval has some mannequin deliver the lines, which closer approximates than a human being the idea of the modern actor. A more accurate description of this illusory actor would be a figure modeled out of raw meat with nervous system laid bare rather than a Surrealist dummy stuffed with sawdust. This play has no lead roles, and these mannequins perform against a backdrop that is real, animated, and, given current norms, formally untheatrical. Thus it entirely rests on words. Yet these words are not expressions or devices to propel the plot forward, they are instruments for creating imaginary tableaux independent of the plot itself, which in precisely calculated time sequences careens toward conclusion, to the ultimate *curtain fall*. The characters, therefore, are not the bearers of these imaginary tableaux because they do not carry the drama. The language of the play is simple, unvarnished, demotic, a language *commonly spoken*. This language is *appalling*, and only this *appalling* language fits the play. The *rhythm* of speech is another element, and Nezval's rhythmic lines show how gratuitous and deceitful the movements of an arm, the dramatic bearing of an actor, the looks pregnant with meaning, and how disgusting and pathetic all those thespian accoutrements such as makeup and wigs.

I believe this drama, which was evidently written as an experiment, will remain foundational for a new era of playwriting. The tension produced by this oddity lies in the relationship between the naturalness of the language and the unpredictable movements that torment the spectator's imagination, by which the actual action is transposed onto the audience where the sounds of sobbing, shrieking, and fainting must necessarily echo if those for whom the play is truly intended are to watch this performance of absolute theater.

Nezval has also discovered objects that have been prematurely discarded : he is working with real things again, and, having swapped out those tawdry and monstrous pasteboard sets of the modern stage, he lets them perform as if he would gladly replace decoration with sections of actual garden and dirt, shrubs, and greenhouse while forgoing both professional and amateur actor, who really don't have any reason to be here.

Nezval's *Fear* is an appalling play, and I cannot think of a more appalling actor than the child who fires a gun. Yet to let a child perform this — and it absolutely *must be* a child — suggests the breeding of a future generation of murderers.

Richard Weiner, *Lazebník* [The Barber], Aventinum, Prague, 1929

Richard Weiner writes in *The Barber :* "Nothing is more compelling than the nakedness of things, and nothing more aloof than a thought, that is, a judgment, that is, what someone thinks about something." I would like to especially remind the initials "tt" in the weekly *Čin* [Action] (no. 22) of these words. Trying to cast himself in the most interesting light possible, this soi-disant "reader (and reviewer)" has made a feeble attempt in brilliantly idiotic diction to pick apart this magnificent book. Who cares? Richard Weiner is a great *modern* poet. Reading his book is akin to recalling the foreign stages on which we should've performed, the foreign journeys from which distance and the course of life have separated us. It is understandable that this type of poetics will never be popular with the denizens of the Powder Tower or the Café Tůmovka.[22] The atmosphere and creatures Weiner creates are *dark,* as dark as certain regions of poetry's future. His prose has a power that is palpable while seeking nothing, representing nothing, and with no *evident reason* for existing. Firemen do not naturally appear at evening to clean their helmets.

The modern poet creates a work that fortunately no one can ravage. Similar in many ways to the ignored Czech poet Jakub Deml, Richard Weiner finds in his works of prose (the song has always preceded the poem just as poetry has historically preceded

[22] Streetwalkers were known to loiter around the Powder Tower; the Tůmovka was a renowned literary café prior to WWI and during the interwar period.

prose) repose in the eternal void, discovering in them the true purpose of dreams. He scorns the musicality of words, the Kralice Bible, stylistic virtuosity, and the perennial fetters of poetry — he knows that some stories need to be divested of their luster because we love them all the more without the sheen. Exhibitionism is only one facet of the malady we might call *joie de vivre*. And this is all the more reason why we should pay attention to those sensations interred in human forms, cloaked in the robes of Judas, and borrowing the wings of angels.

Roman Jaworski, *Svatba hraběte Orgaza* [The Wedding of Count Orgaz], trans. from Polish by F. Bicek, Družstevní práce, Prague, 1930

This novel from "the frontier of two realities," as its subtitle states, is one of the most beautiful translations published by DP. So it is of some interest that because it received so few positive votes from subscribers its publication was relegated to Living Books Editions B.[23] Increasingly absurd incidents and a dramatic ending define the largely extraneous plot. Infinitely more interesting — besides the American millionaire hypnotized by the gaze of Don Fernando Niño de Guevara from El Greco's famous portrait and the prima ballerina Donna Evarista, who falls in love with a bull — is the polymorphic concoction of ideas, observations, dada, sorrow, symbols, meditations, surrealism, problems, etc. that fills the novel.

23 The novel was originally published in Polish as *Wesele hrabiego Orgaza* (1925). The publishing house Družstevní práce was established in 1922 as a cooperative of readers, writers, and artists based on a subscription model. The members voted on the books to be published in the flagship series Živé knihy [Living Books], with the number of votes determining the print run. That this book was consigned to the "B" category implies a rather low print run.

On Painting

Many have tended to reproach us for their inability to understand our paintings. Perhaps it is because lawns release green aniline during a rainstorm that then runs down the slope into the lake. The only curious thing is that the mole avoids cemeteries. — When Lucheni[24] murdered the Austrian Empress, he said : "I killed her because she does no work." Remy de Gourmont adds : "Apparently he killed this woman, who was staying at Lake Geneva incognito, because she was not washing her own clothes." — Any art that comes into being out of hunger or out of a desire for an audience is bullshit. One day humans will reach a stage where we'll be able to reveal the maximum beauty in things. The sun, for example, bakes the rocks before our eyes. But this is only an exchange of relative reality for illusion. Eventually you become accustomed to any *sovereignty* of life. Your friends coalesce with balustrades as proof that forms are transient. The human bee replaces dreams with a mental state that could be called industrious life. If we wouldn't always assume that *certain* memories cannot be recalled without a dose of amnesia, we'd arrive at an art that Eugène Carrière said was supreme, since it speaks to matters in the way we've been taught to understand them. We might vividly imagine the idiots of today who reproach us for creating incomprehensible paintings even *back then* speaking through the mouth of Carrière.

To put it crudely, in nature's embrace we recognized how unjust we've been to ourselves. We came to learn of the poverty of those who could depict a forest without having grasped it. We *observed* that the mauve perfume Klára reeked of was more appalling than the moonlight. After all, the poison that evaporated off her as she slept, so that come morning she could beguile with her innocence, was absorbed by the walls of this room, papered in mist. (She later took this poison abroad concealed in her ginger wig.) Yet back to that morning. By the light of the rising sun Klára walked through the garden with an open knife and cut roses. Time, taking on sun, lent

[24] Italian anarchist Luigi Lucheni (1873–1910) assassinated Austrian Empress Elisabeth in 1898 by stabbing her to death.

naturalness to the scene. Thus far it seems everything has been clear and intelligible to the attentive reader. It should be obvious from the preceding lines, however, that this is mainly about a date pit. We recently read somewhere that an entire archipelago in the Aegean Sea sprang up from the pit of a date. I believe it went something like this : Polynices was hoarding nuts, and a small castle fell out one of them. It got snagged among some reeds in the middle of a lake. P. and I traveled by steamboat around the castle. A moorhen was laying eggs into the castle, and P. was sitting on the eggs. We brought strawberries to keep her from dying of hunger. When moorhen chicks hatched, we put the small castle back into the nut and never shot waterfowl again. Then the curtain fell, and the eyes of a random observer turned everything into desert. The fool painter tried to color in birds on the branches, birds lamenting over not being allowed to step into the jaws of higher order animals.

A time enabling an unbroken chain of surprises has yet to arrive. *Those who seek refuge in sleep are discommoded by having to wait until weariness shuts their eyes.* Certain forms of flowers and human entrails have brought us to meditation, but we did not allow giant models to be constructed from them. We always told Klára : Your head is like a carrot. If you're good, you'll see many different landscapes, but we're still not sure if we'll allow you to enter any of them.

Brief Prolegomena

> *The dialectic of Marx, being the last word in the scientific-evolutionary method, forbids the isolated, i.e., one-sided and abnormally distorted, consideration of an object.*
>
> Lenin

> *If Don Quixote tilts his lance at windmills, that is in accordance with his office and his role; but it would be impossible for us to allow Sancho Panza anything of the sort.*
>
> Engels

> *All that exists, all that lives on land and underwater, exists and lives only by some kind of movement.*
>
> Marx

Autumn once more, the time when the poet takes the harpoon down from the wall and goes out to hunt mermaids. Greetings, blue stockings, continue to dream your dreams of eternal feast!

It depends on you alone if we deem taking a morning tram a matter of need or of entertainment. Once, when I was young, I made the acquaintance of Miss Melusine before I knew how to tell the difference between oats and wheat : Tereza smelled of roses, Aninka of cinnamon, and Kateřina of violets.

The concerns of poetry have never been as simple as they are today. Apart from poets, anyone could decide poetry's future. Gone is the time when poets chose their prince themselves. Gone are those marvelous days when two men would meet in a forest clearing to settle their differences with cudgels. Gone forever are the days when one could display in public a rival's scalp on his belt.

Poets, for the most part, are fools. They're content with rubbing against maidens when they could be triumphing over singing cows. Thanks to their table company, they create immortal works.

One evening the poet met Heraclitus.

Everything simultaneously exists and doesn't exist. Everything flows, everything is constantly changing, everything is always coming into being and coming to an end.

Yes, I understand and know where you're headed with this, the poet replied, but I stand apart from the class struggle for the simple reason that I do not consider myself exploited. No one in the world can steal the fruits of my labor. And if my sympathies do incline toward the working class, it is . . .

Regrettably, Kateřina interrupted, it is also because the cultural needs of the proletariat can be satisfied by a well-chosen turn of phrase.

Dear ladies, Heraclitus remarked, whoever among you states at the outset that she is speaking as a Marxist might have license to sermonize on anything at all.

No one is easier to get drunk than a poet, and the cheapest way is on violet perfume. Poetry will remain *modern* as long as it doesn't pick a fight with the new worldview. Then the Constructivists will make a roundabout return to where they originated. It seems the entire so-called crisis of the working-class intelligentsia lies in the fact that this class was late in grasping the principle of movement, and they reduced the world to a storehouse of things and props while the perpetual merging of events into a straight line and the movement of matter completely escaped their notice. Poetry also became idiosyncratic : via decay, dread, and death. Yet the poet will experience success only when he quits shocking the public.

This is all well and good, said Aninka, I, too, will open myself up to you and spill my guts.

Aninka, perform hara-kiri while seated. And then return to the cemetery dirt soaked with the piss of drunkards and stuff the flora of your bowels back inside you.

As soon as the poet is cognizant of his intents he ceases to be a poet.

One needs to be absolutely clear so that we may speak about what is commonly left unsaid. The issues of poetry have never been as simple as they are today. Poetry's *modernity* is being decided by a handful of students, the random lawyer sticking his iron in the fire of literary criticism at the most opportune moment to attract attention,[25] or those bank clerks occasionally giving their two cents worth on poetry to show how their souls seethe.

Leave them their self-importance, said Tereza, smelling of rose, leave them their delusions that they're creating something while still having demolished nothing. Indulge them and let them write and harangue and judge poetry under the guise of a materialistic worldview. They would become philistines before you mange to have a discussion with them, and such a discussion could only be their gain and your loss. Leave them to observe life through the glass of cafés, from your stomping ground.

The philistine thus far has been of the opinion that everything in nature is modeled on a sphere. The grandiose pebbles of Brâncuși are the closest modern art has ever come to approximating the concepts of eternity and immortality. Only art and poetry that correspond to the level of the proletariat might be called the poetry of the future.

Yet I am destroying myself on purpose, said the poet. I look in the mirror and see myself without makeup, without aureole, without lilies, in such a wretched state that I do not doubt for a second that I in fact resemble a coalman. I know it's not a false likeness because I don't look at myself with *my* eyes.

You see, Kateřina interjected, one day the proletariat will love and admire you. For the meanwhile, what bothers them is that *you still exist*.

If I understand this correctly, Heraclitus said, the poet is not disputing dialectical materialism, nor is he vilifying the proletariat. Rather, he scorns and spits on those Marxist sluggards and their phraseologists, on those abortive scions flushed out the sewers of bourgeois families, on those attenuated revolutionary spirits, on those proletsnobs and communist landlords whom Engels called vulgarizing valets.

If those of inferior mind devote themselves to a philosophical system, they will become *intellects*.

Fellowship and affiliation to a particular class organize their path through life and facilitate their understanding of the dogma that would destroy them as individuals. The Marxist conception of the revolutionary in the context of the dictatorship of the

25 In other words, Ivan Sekanina (see note 18).

proletariat does not, however, controvert the notion that a good revolutionary might be a total dimwit. In any case, how a democrat or a proletarian lolls on a plush divan is of little interest to the poet.

The poet has the right to hide behind an array of faces, said Tereza. The worth of everything that exists is in its eventual annihilation, whispered Mephisto, hiding behind Goethe. Without wood there would be no woodcuts.

The poet is not interested in the question if the ranks of the working class can produce a good poet, as the naissance of a poet-proletarian is nothing exceptional.

Proletarian literature is a successful attempt to rationally lower the intellectual level of the working class. This treachery is being perpetrated on them by virtue of several semi-educated windbags from the most louche margins of society having arrogated the right to satisfy the proletariat's cultural needs. If you look at the world through a Marxist's eyes, what you considered so important before now seems utterly petty and practically worthless, and what you previously deprecated now carries the greatest possible value. It depends on your priorities whether you become a snob or remain a poet, observed Kateřina.

The only thing I care about, the poet replied, is that I'm not identified with those notorious intellectuals from the spring crisis of the intelligentsia that followed on the heels of the conference that was so much like a veterans convention.[26]

It would seem only the deranged and bemused will uphold the tradition of poetry in the future.

Poetry's importance in one's life will be minimal. A poet will have only kin for readers. Marxists are aware of how useless poetry is and that poetry as such, or what we presently imagine to be poetry, is a manifestation of the old world.

26 The Second Conference of Revolutionary Writers held at the end of 1930 in Kharkov, Ukraine, established the hardline communist position on the creation of "proletarian literature and art." Louis Aragon, one of the French delegates at the Conference, duly quit the Surrealist Group early the following year in support of this position and in opposition to Breton's view that so-called "proletarian" literature and art were presently not possible (as he stated in the "Second Manifesto"). Likewise, the Czechoslovak delegates, Vladimír Clementis and Bedřich Václavek, began to write in the early months of 1931 blistering attacks against the avant-garde, thus provoking a great deal of consternation among left-leaning artists.

Let the poet take solace in the fact that today and in the days to come each and every person will rot and disintegrate into dust.

Tereza was the only one who never asked the poet why he put that color in the middle of the square and why he chose such an impenetrable metaphor. Why the brier rose has five petals and why the brier rose even exists, when nothing would change if it did not exist, are questions that do not interest Tereza.

Poetry might be nothing more than those sensations and states superfluous to human existence. One person longs to leave paradise while another longs to enter it.

One disdains the commonplace, another disdains the supernatural. One sees the future of poetry from the outside, another from the inside. The Five-Year Plan neglected to mention how imagination should be regulated. I'm afraid I've become rather decrepit, said the imp from the dark alley. I would look ludicrous if I put any flower other than a red carnation in my buttonhole.

And yet he also loved poetry once, said Aninka, and giving a cryptic smile she straightened her bra.

Silence, Aninka, there was a time when everything was understood as art : shoe shining, confectionery, and in time we shall also cultivate the declining art of burying the dead.

Poetry is merely an opportunity and invitation to dream. In poetry, as in dream, *time* is preserved, the *epoch* buried.

An Inspired Illustrator

An ice cube lay in the shade like a piece of dirty glass. It glinted from piercing sunlight and then melted, sparkling intensely in a conflagration of refracting rays. Having reached a *state of radiance,* it vanished. Real and imagined forms, poetry and fables, are captured and portrayed in Toyen's book illustrations in this *state of radiance*. They vanish and become invisible as *objects* to reappear transformed into arabesques and a tantalizing mélange of points, lines, and planes. Words and the ambience of poetry are recast in pictorial form.

There are two types of reader. One type remains detached from the book even though they conscientiously read each page, filtering the story through their own tastes, comparing the drift of a book to their own worldview, and exploring the psychology of the story by identifying with the characters. All the same, a book might occupy their thoughts for so long that it becomes their best friend. They are conscious readers, stereotypical readers, pillars of culture. They require a reliable illustrator who faithfully reproduces what they are reading. An illustrator who doesn't distress them. An illustrator who has at the ready tried-and-true *clichés* for any subject matter.

Yet this type of illustrator portrays a lover from *The Letters of a Portuguese Nun* in the same way as one of the *Three Musketeers*.

The antithesis of the conscious reader is the reader for whom poetry is a *passion*. A fanatic. The passionate reader is the equal of the poet. A bibliophile who will buy books even during the greatest economic crisis ever. This type doesn't buy books out of a desire for edification, and adores only those illustrations that underpin the thrill that shudders through him without paralyzing his *creative* relationship to reading. *Inspired* illustration.

The inspired illustrator is captivated more by the poet's personality and the work's atmospherics than by extrinsic fabulation, pretentious gesture, and literary genre. If I were to diagram the position of the inspired graphic artist it would be as the point where two lines — one representing the character of the poet and the other the character of the work — figuratively intersect.

Illustration should echo the reader's emotions. Toyen's illustrations are a wager in the *game* of reading. There is never a discrepancy between the content and creative collaboration in the books she has illustrated. Her drawings stir and augment our imagination, which no matter how autonomous and rich in and of itself can never escape the hold her work has on it. It's as if we were marked by her gossamer drawings that go beyond the beginning and end of a story to stay embedded in our minds. So it happens that we encounter the eyes of J.K. Tyl's Malcontent[27] on the low wall of a village tavern at the height of summer somewhere in Bavaria, and we will no longer be able to think of him without his amorous gaze upturned toward the emptiness and darkness as the whole of his past.

Toyen's drawings have managed to fill in part of the universe of modern humanity. These curious, artificial, and yet compact drawings, which she has attained through a *unified* evolution, harbor the absolute power of evocation within their succinct and precise idiom. In the perpetual melding of analogies with identical real forms, of memories having no definitive shape with grim naturalistic imagery, visualized between the lines of poetry and in allusions overlaying pregnant descriptions, she captures above all the poet and his stories from places we were not in the habit of seeing.

So for Joseph Delteil's terrible Don Juan legend she created an analogous subject who suffers, introducing ubiquitous chaos and horror. She created those unspeakable *predestinations of the grave*. How could we ever forget that ecstatic and putrid face, which will accompany us along the cemetery walls and always be with us whenever our thoughts turn to our *future*. For it is our supreme likeness.

When reading *The Heptameron,* that extravagant collection of tales in a constant state of flux, we become cognizant of the giant reservoir of human characters, and when we compare the book's atmosphere with the copious drawings created by Toyen,

[27] Josef Kajetán Tyl (1808–56) published his novella *Rozervanec* [The Malcontent] in 1840 in the magazine *Vlastimil*. One of the characters is named Hynek, an allusion to Karel Hynek Mácha and vehicle for Tyl to deride Mácha's adoption of the Byronic malcontent as something alien to the Czech spirit. Tyl also authored the Czech national anthem "Kde domov můj?"

we see that the choice of illustrator could not have been more apt. Toyen has succeeded in creating a type of modern erotic illustration. Her drawings reveal a single indulgence : the relish for a young girl's beauty. The torsos of women, exalted eyes full of amorous boredom, horrifying and twisted at the moment of orgasm, tenderly misted in the hour of death, breasts veiled by a passing cloud, pierced by a dagger, the shade of a girl's sex covered by a stray piece of lace, the gesture of hands on a cushion, untied bodice strings, the lecherous mouth of an itinerant monk, a graceful leg, a nude maiden's shoulder tilted over a sleeping boy, and the entire repertoire of unctuous details constituting the game of love. Only when our eyes wander the contours of this world of women, many times *clad* only in a smile, are we able to dream to the full intensity of the stories in *The Heptameron,* which depict in such singular fashion life's highs and lows.

The Joys of a Book Illustrator

Does anyone mock a mermaid because she has no legs? I tell you, a terrible era of visionaries and meditation is on the horizon, an era similar to the time immediately preceding Creation. Men will love tree trunks and women will be born who resemble Venus with the allegorical faces of sedulity, nobility, verity, and beauty. New Judiths will emerge out of eternity and immortality and drive to the slaughterhouse, through the city streets lined with onlookers, a herd of paunchy cattle who look at the demolished monuments with the disappointed eyes of demiurges. Cows in bandages with severed legs will graze in the parks and city gardens as their prostheses trample the green lawns. Poets will stroll in this sultry atmosphere stinking of phenol and point out to the random reader of the evening news the beauty of creating. Painters will cut their canvases into smaller pieces and no one will count them and no one will notice that they once formed a single whole. It will be an era of air, water, land, and fire blending slowly, an era that will see the dreamed-of synthesis of material and lyrical beauty. Animals will freely interbreed, and new unicorns and insect-mammals, fabulous rams, and creatures constructed from blades, needles, and daggers, creatures made of cotton wool, snakeskin, plumed trees, animal-like creatures glued together from the immortal works of poets and from flowerpots, and many other obscene monsters, all will come into being outside the supervision of biologists.

All that is left for us is to begin anew following the lead of little Bosko and create new stories from old themes, while the society of the fêted, as a way to avoid their natural inclination to imitate, will revise our aesthetic concepts. As has been the case from time immemorial, a new poetry and a new art will be born of desire, that nothing the poet experiences will fall into oblivion : from vanity and from selflessness, from self-aggrandizement, avarice, betrayal, courage, and from curiosity, from an inferiority complex and a sovereignty of the spirit, because a person is both good and evil, because a person loves and hates, and because we shall always remain clowns in prudent society.

O how perspicacious you were, dear wife of Verlaine, when you forbade him absinthe. You forbade him from drinking the stuff lest certain ideas come into his head.

The illustration is commonly a synthesis of readers' impressions. Metaphorically stated, the contents of one vessel poured into another of different shape. Just recall the bogus contortions of literal graphic art whereby notions of melancholy, tragedy, pathos, coquetry and so forth are trotted out in *visual form* while so fastidiously adhering to the *poetic style!*

To require the illustrator to express sorrow wherever the poet exhibits sorrow is misguided. When the poet and the illustrator coincide, the result is caricature. For the true lover of poetry, the pictorial expression of verbal metaphors and synonyms is a distraction. An inferior illustrator approaches the work with the joint ambition to be a servant to the poet, the darling of readers, and a hit for the publisher. No illustration, save kitsch, is ever able to convey the idea of the work.

Modern illustration accentuates the relationship between the *principle* of the work and its *formal expression*. It fills the nonfigurative space that arises during a reader's reveries and in the fantasies that linger after the actual act of reading. The modern illustration naturally adapts to the intention of the poetic work while retaining its own independent existence. The *thematic* dimension of the poetic work concurs with the *subject* of the illustration, and vice versa.

What are readers of Ovid's *Tristia* left with besides fragments of troubled thoughts, wanderings, a cluster of words and places, images and wigs, gnawed bones, a gardening apron and sewer pipes, central heating, memories of a steamboat on the Danube, and the desire to rifle through Goethe's luggage?

The Painter Who Draws : Man with a Flaming Mane!

Painters do not like to exhibit their drawings. They have their reasons, it seems, for keeping their sketches hidden. Emil Filla is one of those painters who does exhibit them. A good drawing brings out the inner life of the painter. It is an explosion of his unconscious, created in a trance-like state. It is akin to the painter delivering a soliloquy. In Filla's opening remarks to his exhibition *Beautiful Chamber* (January–February, 1933) he eloquently stated : "drawing is a most intimate affair when depicting and incarnating one's ideas. It is a dialogue between the artist and nature, but a dialogue that of necessity turns into the artist's monologue."

Drawing should not be profaned through exposition as its strength lies in inspired silences and exuberant shorthand, all of which bear witness to the presence of a poet. Filla's drawings are created in a trance, that is, in a state when the painter is more poet than visual artist. They can neither be judged as documentation of his creative method nor as aids for the execution of his paintings. That would understate them. They should be appreciated as the purest form of modern artistic expression because they exhibit all the signs of a great work. They undermine our expectations. Filla's fusion of realistic observations with the lineaments of dreams stimulates our interest in plain and magical things and forms we have long forgotten. As draftsman, Filla creates the illusion that we are experiencing his afternoons, and in this way he tells us about places, summer, the music of wings, and time without depicting anything or anyone outside himself. And yet in his drawings fruit ripens pungently, forests of Swedish matches burn, lead weights melt, and wax faces disintegrate. His drawings limn a *Paradise of Things.*

His creative mode is growth, or better said, the evolution of one form from another, not their alternation : His grapes spoke with the sun. Not everyone is able to enjoy the most sublime creations of the human spirit. Thus very few understand the language of his glasses. If I had to find an analogy for Filla's drawings in poetry, I might mention Cocteau's delightfully abbreviated lines or Aragon's improvisations. Scorning the artistic demands of the public, these poets created their work for a handful of peers scattered, unfortunately, over great distances, although luckily in all corners of the world. Several of Filla's drawings have no parallel in the whole of modern art. The person who knows the *actual* state of European art and perceives beauty more than philosophizes about it will be able to appreciate in Filla's drawings his striking and expansive individuality, which is not a repetition of inventiveness or of someone hermetically closed off.

Alas, imbeciles have the final say in our society, and critics and public opinion are increasingly coming to resemble, as old Pascal would say, a sphinx with the head of an ass. May this creature continue to graze on the pretty aniline green fields of Czech landscape painting.

Flashback : Toyen's Spring Postcards

I remember one evening years ago in Sanary, a seaside village near Toulon, Toyen and I were sitting in the front yard of a café under a tree, the botanic name of which escapes me, but it lives in my memory under the moniker *silver plane with bearded balls*. It was February. Spring. No breeze. The air saturated with the smell of fish fried in oil, and the sea a pale shade of gray, only a school of rowboats gently rocking on it, speaking in whispers. Behind the wall of a house, set against the sky, a dense web of pine (?) branches. And it was on this road leading to the cemetery that Derain had set up his easel. It is his landscape after a rainstorm with clouds rent and the giant trunks . . . (of what?).

We talked about spring in Bohemia, and while we were talking Toyen absentmindedly drew on the green tin table surface breasts, snowdrops, cats, lilies of the valley, a girl's eye, tree buds, a bird in front of a birdhouse, and all sorts of other figures I cannot begin to enumerate! I only remember that eventually it became a medley of forms, one intruding on the next, forms dissolving into an indistinguishable arabesque, an ingenious scrawl.

When I first saw Toyen's series of springtime drawings on the postcards published by Družstevní práce, I thought back to that evening in Sanary. I think it was then, in that distant place, this Bohemian spring was born, the origin of these incomparable drawings on that tabletop scrawl in the café we left like delinquents under the reproachful eye of the proprietor.

Toyen has the rare gift to evoke remote memories in the sensitive viewer. Through well-calculated line, point, glint in the eye, the simplest means, she manages to titillate the most complex states, to touch the viewer in the most sensitive spots and at the most impressionable moments. This is the ground for the sophisticated manner in which she has composed the gradual transition from winter to spring, that *most tantalizing* season of the year, when earth and rain are redolent, when the faces of young girls are still carefree and innocent, their hands groping in space. It is the time of year when star clusters quiver, when the mornings are cool, and the chirping of nestlings is heard at dawn. It is a spring that isn't yet a *bazaar of kisses*. Modern, artistically conceived and imagined, this series of drawings depicting the ambience of early spring in Bohemia bears the stamp of memory and of a lengthy creative gestation, a long period of crystallization.

The Landscape of Marquis de Sade

History is nothing if not the remarkable dissipation of truth in time. This is why the names of poets are always connected to ruins and shadows. Everything the poet forsakes turns gray and becomes ash. Poets delight in observing how oblivion corrupts the forms of what was once beauty, how emptiness expands in hearts once vital, how everything around them ripens toward death, how everything rushes toward expiration, while their hearts are denied the benevolence of aging. Todays and tomorrows are not a poet's concern, time is.

The Marquis de Sade, one of the greatest minds and the literary paragon of the 18th century, escaped, fortunately, the notice of his contemporaries. — His extensive oeuvre has only received its proper due today, and his proscribed name, shrouded for the whole 19th century by heinous legend, only now has been completely rehabilitated.

The sky, azure as the distance, arches over his landscape. I passed through in summer so that I could brush its horizons, read the collapsed walls of La Coste, and later reliably isolate from the bare brown earth of its vineyards on the Saumane slopes that tint of blood lying more than a hundred years on the memory of him.

The ruins of Castle La Coste are located far from the main arteries between Avignon and Apt. The countryside around it is arid, rocky, and plaintive even in the blazing noonday sun, when the pebbles on the road are white and the grape leaves hot. It is quiet, and the fragrance of thyme accompanies the fool trekking through the broom. Yet at evening the light recedes into rose, and the entire landscape takes on the exuberant air of a cabaret. The clouds begin to slow their course, and a peculiar violet hue burgeons in the distance, one that does not recur beyond this part of Provence and is perceived only by the most sensitive eye accustomed to remembering the dead, a hue passing right into dreams and coloring them with this taboo impression of evil. The bare moon, its light piercing the deep darkness of the branches, brings sleep to the indolent and, compelling lovers to aimlessly wander the countryside, drives the lunatic from this demonic paradise.

So it was here, at night, that I invoked the shade whose true likeness was never captured, the shade dashing off on a gimpy horse over the low vineyard walls and across the fields headed south, toward Marseille, while in the distance on the castle's terraces the torches gutter out and an assemblage of dishabilled Lyon tarts belts out lewd songs.

Few castles in 18th-century Provence could compare with the magnificence and splendor of this favorite residence of Marquis de Sade. His coat of arms was carved above the gates : a black eagle in a gold star, the family motto, *Sade toujours,* inscribed underneath.

Sade had Castle La Coste renovated to be an occasional residence for him and his wife. But when their already tepid relationship turned frigid, and she preferred Château de Saumane, he lived here alone surrounded by a coterie of drunkards and girls. There is no other place on earth, save the prisons at Miolans, Pierre-Encise, Vincennes, and the Bastille, in which Sade spent a total of twenty-seven years, more closely associated with his name than this piece of ground where he lived the fullest moments of his life in freedom.

A beautiful dancer and singer by the name of Beauvoisin, to whom he referred as his wife, was now living with him. She was slim, perhaps suffering from consumption, and she was a redhead. To make her feel at home at La Coste, Sade had her room painted with obscene tableaux. Let's have no illusions about this petite singer and dancer from the 18th century. Did she sit barefoot on the north wall? Did she dance on the terraces in the shadows of the setting sun? Did she resemble an ancient priestess with bluish lips? Let's have no illusions about love!

It takes only one conversation for two hearts to become forever estranged, one second for lovers to slip forever from each other's embrace.

Castle La Coste is the only place we can associate with love in Marquis de Sade's life. One day his sister-in-law, Louise de Montreuil, paid him a visit. She was the only love of his life. Fair-haired, her smile ignited Sade's forebodings. A spring breeze rustled the olive groves on the castle's slopes. Louise loved the garden's dark, damp recesses. Shadow followed the angel. And when the Marquis first pressed her translucent hand, she fainted and fell face first to the ground. It was spring in Provence, and for no one was Saint-Just's later pronouncement more apt : "The milk of liberty! 'tis blood."

While the Marquis was making ready to abscond with Louise to Italy, redheaded Beauvoisin, reminiscing, languished in the arms of a shady lawyer who had set up shop in the passageway of the Palais-Royal — she was subsequently swept from the ranks of the living by the wave of revolution.

No place on earth reminds me more of a graveyard than the ruins of La Coste washed with sun. Louise as well would never see her paramour's region again. She died the following year in Venice, execrated by her family but in the Sade's arms. Whoever wallows in the void does not make a keepsake of fallen hairpins. The Marquis de Sade was not one to look back.

Castle La Coste was deserted. Grass grew on the tiled terraces, nettles filled the nooks, and dirt accumulated in the cellars.

Then the French Revolution happened. One morning a mob broke into the castle of the hated aristocrat, plundered it, and set it ablaze. To this day people in the region still claim that subterranean chambers were found with the most terrible instruments of torture and piles of human bones. This might very well be one of the sources for the horrific Sade legend. The detailed report on the castle's pillage, now housed in the archives of the Conseil National of Apt, gives no evidence that anything of the sort was ever discovered. Even so, there is mention of a "room with immoral scenes" and a "hall with paintings depicting the most varied uses of an enema," in short, nothing shocking to anyone in the 18th century.

The Marquis de Sade learned of his home's destruction while imprisoned at Picpus in Paris, and soon thereafter he sold the castle and its grounds to Deputy of Parliament Rovère, who came to open the doors of the jail for him. Ownership has changed hands many times since, but the castle's buildings have never been rebuilt. This is all well and good. It would be an inexcusable act of vandalism to deny time its nourishment.

Today the extensive ruins blend in with the sporadically inhabited settlement of ramshackle houses below it. A small lizard suns itself on a dirty white stone of the wall. A tricolored cat sleeps nearby. A large black butterfly with yellow spots floats over a

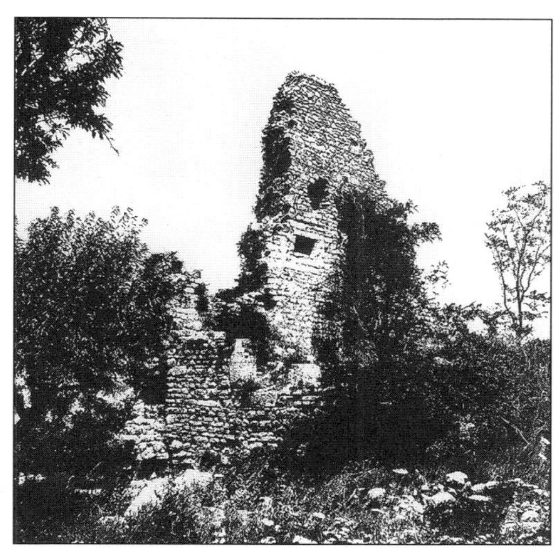

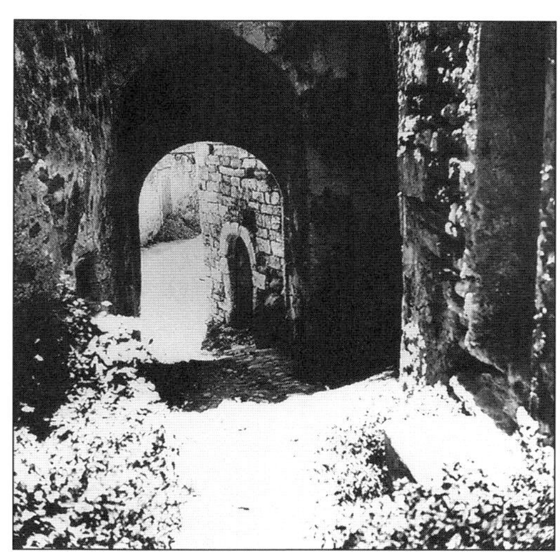

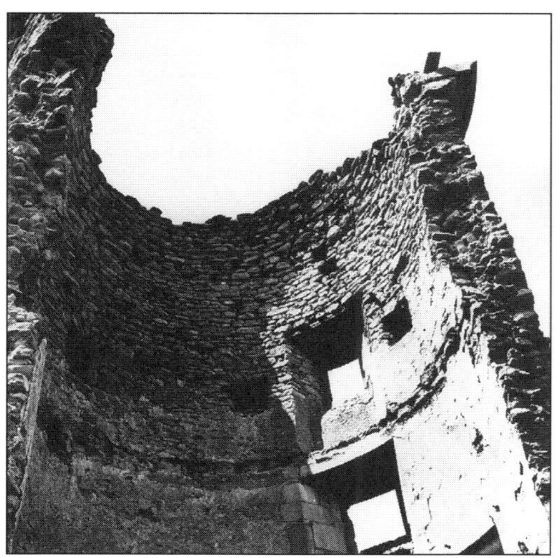

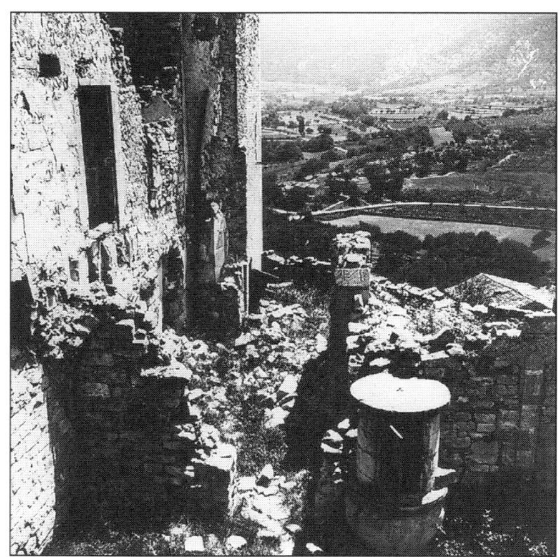

child's white shirt drying in the sun. Woodworms tirelessly work on the remains of the heavy gates, the disused knocker having rusted. Ivy, moss, and mold cover the walls jutting skyward with their derelict window openings. In a quiet corner overgrown with geraniums a gray marble hearth is crumbling. Here the remnants of subtly modeled plaster flowers and fine moulding still linger on the walls darkly saturated with an orange hue, a kind of mix of vermilion and yellow that will never vanish from my memory. It is a particularly noxious color that always came to mind when reading *Maldoror*.

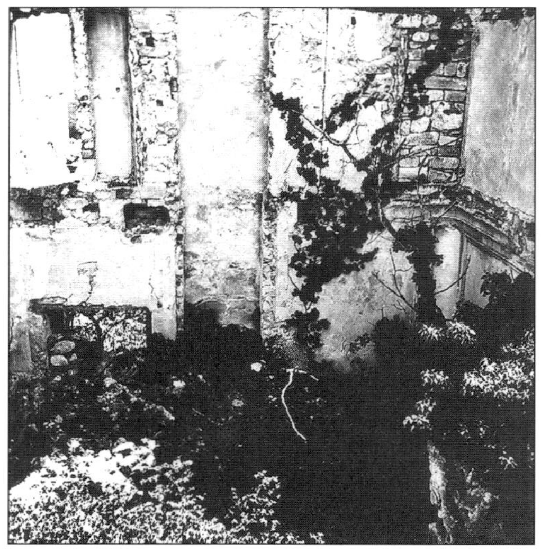

Surrealist Painting

(a few observations)

Someone with a disposition that André Breton has called Surrealist, a Surrealist poet or painter for whom spontaneity is process, will be (without having to explain this process) in complete accord with the observations of dialectical materialism, which is not a bogus doctrine and is based on observing the laws of objective being. If the spontaneity of the poet or the painter is indeed automatic, and they would like to explain their work only on the basis of intuition without any philosophical pretensions, I think they will ultimately come to the conclusion that the perspective of dialectical materialism must be considered self-evident. When it comes to the spontaneity I'm speaking about, Salvador Dalí has recently put it rather nicely : "All these considerations lead me to be generally suspicious of 'spontaneity' in its pure state, in which I always recognize the conventional and stereotyped taste of the invariable restaurant crayfish, and personally to prefer, rather than spontaneity, 'systematization' which, like paranoiac delirium, can occur and in fact does occur 'spontaneously' . . ."[28]

I would like to ground this brief analysis exclusively in such intuition. I leave its validation to the gnoseology of dialectical materialism, which, knowing the exact laws of reality and objective being, illuminates, as applied in psychology, even the most subtle facets of thought processes positivism could never explain and idealism has stood on their head.

As long as I was at odds with dialectical materialism, as long as I hadn't thoroughly integrated its perspective, I never considered if what is called semblance had its concrete basis in the laws of actual being. The aesthetics of Artificialism differed from the gnoseology of Surrealism in that they did not call into question the reality of semblance. In practice, the intuition of the painter, spontaneously requiring this connection to a real core, was, it seems to me, reliable enough so as not to contradict

28 In *Dalí on Modern Art: The Cuckolds of Antiquated Modern Art*, Salvador Dalí, tr. Haakon M. Chevalier (New York: The Dial Press, 1957).

the laws of objective being, even if interpretation of this practice might too easily have slipped into idealism.

If I had to situate Artificialism, I would call it a link between Cubism and Surrealism. At the time Surrealism was in its incipiency in France there were no Surrealist paintings to speak of. Even André Breton considered those painters just coming into his orbit as forerunners more than full-fledged representatives of Surrealist painting. Most of them were already fairly well-defined as artists — Picasso, Chirico, Klee, Arp, Masson, Picabia — and their work was more a reference point for Breton than a basis. But others who essentially were just starting out — Tanguy, Miró, Ernst, Dalí — were lambasted, and not without justification, for adopting an illustrative, literary, anecdotal approach to painting (with the sole exception perhaps of Miró). Today, when the majority of these artists have developed in a way that is evolutionary, save Max Ernst, whose development could be called revolutionary, the situation is different. I preferred to refrain from using any foreign devices in making my shift from Artificialism to Surrealism, and I did not betray my intuition, which guided me, I believe, correctly. It was, however, that intellectual perspective of idealism standing on its head that in due time created discord between myself and some of those folks who were rather rigorously trying to modify their ideology to conform to the position of dialectical materialism.

Surrealism rediscovered for painting reality and its emotive content, which resides in its psychic meaning. The particular appearance of a phenomenon is deeply rooted, that is, if we don't take it as some brilliant piece of ambitious subjectivity. It is rooted in the laws of reality's objective being as viewed from a dialectical and materialistic perspective rather than from a positivistic perspective.

Surrealist painting, therefore, largely mines intuitive knowledge. Yet this is not intuition in the Bergsonian sense, that is, intuition as a form of the immediate experience of superempirical, transcendent, metaphysical reality.

To illustrate how distant we are today from the original idea of Cubism, I refer to Picasso's statement that he wanted to paint in such a way that an engineer would be able to construct the objects depicted in the painting. To quote Dr. Vincenc Kramář :

"Cubism's main concern was form, plasticity, and the precise disposition of things in space, and to depict these elements as objectively as possible. This image of objects would also have other features, such as color, and aspects that we apprehend with highly subjective senses. To fill the picture surface with this profound understanding of things and to bring out their full beauty through the painting's composition, this was the ultimate objective of Picasso and Braque, in other words, of Cubism."[29]

Being aware that art is a process that aims toward producing a higher value through the interplay of contrasts, we salute Cubism for being such a breathtaking, epochal antipode to practically the whole of painting's historical evolution up till tht time. Kramář defined more clearly and accurately than any art critic the historical role of Cubism, which gave birth to Surrealism, which in turn only *ostensibly* denies Cubism's contribution. Only ostensibly. In terms of worldview, Cubism springs from an idealistic conception of artistic form and philosophically links to the theories of Kant and Schiller : "In a truly beautiful work of art the content should do nothing, the form everything" (Schiller). Surrealist painting revives the existence of things. I do not mean to say that Cubism was an entirely abstract art, particularly in its latter phases. We only need to look at the latest works of Picasso and Filla to see this, and only a narrow crevice separates them from Surrealism.

Surrealism regards the relationship between form and content dialectically. Today, after the epochal discoveries of Cubism, the whole fetishizing of so-called pure painting is alien to our thinking, as are all the questions about space and its creation with non-illusionistic means, the question of light, the questions over dissolving the firm contours of solids, the fragmentation of objects into their constituent parts, the natural fears of distortion, atmosphere, illusionism as an impure mode of artistic expression. The Surrealist painter is capricious in the choice and use of plastic means. In the Surrealist painting, form and content are united. Structure and composition are not ends in themselves in the Surrealist painting as they are with "pure painting."

[29] Dr. Vincenc Kramář (1877–1960) was a Czech patron of the arts, collector, and art historian, and one of the leading experts on Cubism. He donated his exceptional collection of Cubist art to the National Gallery in Prague.

Envision, if you will, the Surrealist artist who is painting a swath of unfolding canvas. The Surrealist painter does not create a composition as much as replaces an artificial arrangement with one that has arisen spontaneously, the result of long years of creating composition directed by instinct, an accumulation of experience without being cognizant of it. The Surrealist painting is a response to painting that would like to elicit only an optical impression. Surrealist painting seeks direct and profound psychic expression and as such it is outside the scope of any purely aesthetic evaluation. Surrealist paintings are, as Karel Teige has so aptly put it : "Incendiary flashes of imagination : the imagination that once gave birth to sphinxes, dryads, centaurs, dolphins, harpies, demons, and angels, today creates monsters more strange than a woman's body with the tail of a fish, new sirens far from the representations of women and fish."

Surrealism, the revival of Romanticism.

One final remark : I wish our art critics wouldn't so glibly toss around such labels as *Surrealist painting* and *Surrealist painter,* and would learn to distinguish between those for whom Surrealism is their natural habitat and those who are so adroit at plundering the world of imagination, the imitators and pirates using the idea of Surrealism as cover.

From a lecture given at an evening of the
Surrealist Group at Mánes Gallery,
Prague, May 11, 1934

Surrealist Photography

I have been taking photographs for about fifteen years, and over this time I've shot many, photographically flawless, with the gratification and passion of the card-carrying amateur photographer of today whose formulaic pictures are inundating exhibitions across the world. But none of this interests me anymore. In fact, it bores me.

The only thing about photography that really engages me at present is discovering the surreality concealed in everyday objects. Needless to say, this precludes any sort of aesthetic formalism, which directly subverts Surrealist photography, and it likewise precludes any interest in abstract and lensless photography. *Surrealist photography is not abstract photography.* It is therefore a fundamental misunderstanding to consider the Brno Photogroup of Five[30] Surrealist photography — as the uninformed in our country are wont to think. This group produces nothing but run-of-the-mill aesthetic photography, nourished by an enchantment with Man Ray, Moholy-Nagy, etc.

The genesis of Surrealist photography, as we understand it and you may see for yourself in the Mánes Gallery, is inseparably linked to objects that are passé, keepsake objects, the bizarre, like hairdresser's dummies, artificial legs, and such. These objects harbor a latent symbolism, which the ordinary process of taking a photograph accentuates, making the objects, as V. Nezval has said, "like the ultra-material and virtually ungraspable denizens of dreams." The whole issue with photography is in being prepared to be astonished when coming across a particular object and then to mentally imbue it with surreality. To be sure, chance and being attuned to the object are crucial.

And naturally we will not remain confined to this world of hairdresser's dummies and automatons — which we discovered and have since looked on as they became feed for dilettante photographers — yet our new discoveries are our secret for now. As for technique, our work endeavors to achieve the least possible distortion of subject

30 Fotoskupina pěti, or F5, was an avant-garde photographer collective formed in Brno and active during the interwar period.

matter, whether through the manipulation of light or in how the photograph is taken — the subject should be potent enough to make its presence felt.

The two series of photographs I am exhibiting arose out of the random arrangement of individual photographs whose captions underscore their latent meaning.

The Importance of Emil Filla

The admiration the Surrealists have for Picasso is, among other things, rooted in their recognition of the singular value freedom of expression has in the service of concrete irrationality. Picasso represents the most daring utilization and assertion of inspiration in its most liberated form, and the novelty of its "hybrid creatures" are an ingenious dramatization of concrete irrationality. The superficial, purely mechanical interpretation of Picasso led the era into a most ill-fated, pointless fallacy, and this goes by the name of abstract art. As long as various abstract artists were eager to be labeled with the shaky construct of Cubism, then this construct would remain nothing more than a sweeping generalization of the cubic. So these sundry abstract artists saw in Picasso nothing more than the originator of an epithet that proceeded from his absolute incomprehension and shallow interpretation of the first "cubist" canvases.

We should therefore acknowledge that Emil Filla deserves great credit for being able to realize Picasso's exceptional value during the very early days of his revolution in painting, and likewise for then being able to divorce his concerns from the concerns of the manifold "cubisms," which might seem original in respect to Picasso but in fact are no more original than a magician's worn-out bowler that possesses a mystique they've never had.

It is not hard today to recall the stampede of many of Filla's contemporaries away from the challenge posed by Picasso when this very challenge required of those who took it on a variable and rather firm rectitude when recognizing the risk of being shut out from sale and forgoing the lucrative social standing that official, or at least compromised, art desires. In the end, it was an amusing stampede and, as it could only be, contemptible. Most bolted toward officially sanctioned kitsch, and a few came to a compromise between kitsch and the cube. Emil Filla will always be remembered for making Picasso's concerns fatefully his own with all the deleterious consequences this entailed, thereby setting the cornerstone of a serious and high-minded modernism in the Czech lands. Despite all the concomitant pitfalls, he took the path of intrepid growth over the nearly universal selling out, and thus established the benchmark against which anyone in the future who would like to think himself a creator of an artistic era will have to be measured. By his methodical and principled cultivation of Picasso's concerns in an utterly antiseptic moral milieu, Emil Filla more than anyone else emancipated Czech painting from dilettantism, from its service to the ruling class and popular taste, from the swamp of perpetual compromise and a plethora of options, from mindless opportunism, and from the provincial minding of one's p's and q's. If sacrifice was required, and given the era, Emil Filla had to sacrifice some of the most intimate corners of his unconscious to the path he had chosen, it was recompensed by his art, in all its expressive and structural facets, being elevated to such heights that it serves as guarantee that the quality of Czech painting in the future will never again be allowed to sink to the lows experienced before Filla's radical intervention.

There is little need to highlight the magnificent lyricism pervading Filla's work. And yet it is this lyricism that imbues his work with a quality that is not a Constructivist working out of technical problems but an expression of sensibility that Baudelaire called the definition of life.

Štyrský & Nezval

One who is no longer young . . .

One who is no longer young rids his life of much that is superfluous. He tosses out the ballast. One day he peruses his library and mercilessly discards the books he no longer cares about and knows he'll never read again. And this is what I have done : I have culled my bookshelf of the entire oeuvre of a certain poet whom I shall not name. Yet I do often return to Vítězslav Nezval's work, especially to reread *Poems of Night (The Marvelous Magician), Woman in the Plural, The Jewish Cemetery,* and *The Absolute Gravedigger*. I also reread František Halas. His unforgettable *Gentiana* and *Beautiful Misfortune* will always captivate me. I like Jaroslav Seifert. I consider *On the Waves of TSF* to be his finest volume of poetry. I admire Jindřich Hořejší's "Lady from the Seaside" and Vladimír Holan's *Meridians* and *The Dream*. Of the older poets, I'm fond of *Night of Chimeras* by Viktor Dyk, *My Purgatory* by Jakub Deml, and the work of Karel Hlaváček. *For me the most modern Czech poem is "May" by K.H. Mácha.* — One who is no longer young loves youth. I have read nearly every collection put out by younger poets but have found nothing in them other than convention, verbal musicality, and saccharine verse. These young poets take themselves for militants, yet no one has informed them that they are fighting for something our generation long ago conquered and abandoned. For that matter, today's literary critics seem to me like crazy surveyors who have placed "our Czech spinning wheel" on their geodetic instruments. I know a single young poet, Jindřich Heisler, I know his poems and texts (published by Albert Skira in Paris to accompany Toyen's series of drawings *Les Spectres du désert*), who is the only one at present to have resisted the scent of printer's ink. — Of the foreign poets, I count Paul Eluard, André Breton, and Benjamin Péret as my favorites. *I consider the greatest modern poet of ALL to be Lautréamont* (Les Chants de Maldoror).

Assorted Text Fragments

• THE NIGHT OF APRIL 13-14, 1939

Who's writing to you is not important. It is only a stranger who wishes to express his deep admiration and enchantment. He would like to thank you for the magnificently captivating moment he heard your Marianne and devoured her with his eyes, as his eyes need to be continually fed.

Fortunately words are not his mode of expression. He isn't a poet. But he is someone who imagine's a girl's movement, who dissects horror, the wind, memory, and nothing from the sacks of silliness he sits on escapes him.

Marianne, everything good and evil in life has its source in dreams. Maybe you're familiar with Gérard de Nerval's *Aurélia,* which begins with the words : *Our dreams are a second life.* Maybe you're familiar with his story, which ended so tragically. I, too, have been close to the heart of despair. Life only has the value we give it. It was a product of this disgusting era, treachery everywhere, the arts full of corruption, cowardice, and many other matters of a private nature. Same goes for the air we are obliged to breathe in our so beloved heart of Europe! And then : everything, all I had believed in, was behind me. Irrevocably. It all left me exhausted.

By what magic have you appeared in my life? What strange fate has caused our paths to cross? I don't know whether it was more love or admiration I felt for you. Be at ease, Marianne! I have now overcome my crisis. It's just that reason whispers to me that something more awful than despair is now afoot in the world.

I am ashamed I've revealed so many details. Maybe now you have some idea who has written to you. I implore you never to speak about this. Console me that you didn't recognize me, that you thought it was some idiot who wanted one day to exchange his wretched heart for a replica.

If only I were able to cure myself of life!

I envision Marianne clad in white satin. What a pity it isn't dotted with rowanberries. She is gorgeous. I see her at the footlights, smiling, happy. Reaping applause.

She's a success. Marianne is a *genuine* actress of very high caliber. As Mademoiselle Rachel, Sarah Bernhardt, and Nazim were in their day. What a pity she has come to bury my spring.

Until we meet again at night, I will never be certain you even exist. I will avoid your shadow but will rub elbows with people, prostitutes, and vixens.

Why am I writing you all this? I would like to write a book about you. Too bad I'm not a poet!

- **1939**

Poor woman, though I had patiently endured your moods I finally had to split with you. I couldn't live with so many contradictions. I flew into your life in the guise of a night moth, singed my wings, and then vanished back into the night. I seemed gigantic to you in flight, but after I alighted next to you a few times you became accustomed to seeing me as very small. Those who know me know that I am very, very modest. I am incapable of being rude, especially to women. But they also know I have accomplished everything in my life I've set my mind to. To some folks I've been cruel while gentle with friends and bringing joy to those I like. Consequently, many hate me, yet even those who hate me most cannot begrudge me a certain respect. You will also come to hate me, though you will adore me in a corner of your heart! How I understand you today! Our story began as a drama for the stage. For me it was a dance on a wire, and for you it was a dalliance linked to your desire for a career. I wrote you : "Your drama might be the death of me. Show some mercy!" I managed to stage our piece. We were both healthy, I did not die, and you are celebrating success as a conventional actress in an operetta. I began work on a painting for you, since you once told me my drawings looked like the pictures in *La Vie Parisienne*.[31] And since you kept insisting, I had the following announcement placed in the daily newspaper *Lidové noviny* :

[31] Founded in 1863, *La Vie Parisienne* [Parisian Life] was a French weekly magazine that was hugely popular in the early 20th century and continued to come out without interruption until 1970.

Artist Inspired by Actress

Jindřich Štyrský is working on a series of twelve paintings titled *The Moods of Marianne* after Alfred de Musset's play of the same name, which was staged by D40 with Marie Burešová,[32] the inspiration for Štyrský's series, in the lead role ("Culture Chronicle," *Lidové noviny*, Nov. 24, 1939, p. 7).

- **THE MOODS OF MARIANNE**

The Moods of Marianne is conceived as a composition measuring 150 x 260 cm that comprises twelve 50 x 65 cm paintings set in a single frame, each one of which may be freely rearranged according to "mood." I have asked you to please give me time. My modus operandi is to paint like a poet composes a poem. I believe the painter is greater than the paintings he hides behind. *The Moods of Marianne* will include the inscription : "This greatest burden and most beautiful part of my life I dedicate to the actress Marie Burešová." The following words should be printed when published in book form : *For future psychoanalysts*. The first image was to be of "The Tiny Alabaster Hand";[33] the second "Dream — Humoresque"; the third *"Belle au bois dormant"*;[34] the fourth "Mayakovsky's Vest";[35] the fifth "At Astolaine's Grave";[36] the sixth "Ballad"; the seventh "The Year 1939"; the eighth "Naples"; the ninth "I know no greater

32 *Les Caprices de Marianne* was written by French dramatist Alfred de Musset in 1833; D39, D40, etc. was E. F. Burian's (see note below) experimental theater denoted by D (for *divadlo*) + year of season. Štyrský was involved in a tempestuous affair with the actress Marie Burešová, who appeared in a number of Burian's productions. Three roles performed by Burešová particularly resonated with Štyrský : Marianne in Musset's play (premiere on April 12, 1939); Astolaine (cf. "The Ever-Shrinking World") in Maurice Maeterlinck's marionette drama *Alladine and Palomides* that was adapted into Czech verse by Vladimír Holan (premiere in mid-December 1939, its program illustrated by Štyrský's *Icebound Woman*); and the lead in Vítězslav Nezval's verse adaptation of *Manon Lescaut* (premiere on May 7, 1940).

33 "A Little Hand Made out of Alabaster" is one of Božena Němcová's (1820–62) fairly tales.

34 The classic fairy tale penned by Charles Perrault and known in English as "Sleeping Beauty."

35 Dated December 1939, it was originally inspired by "Marianne" but bears the inscription : "This PIECE of my life I dedicate to Toyen."

36 "Astolaine" was later dropped from the title; see Teige's Introduction.

egomaniac . . ."; the tenth "Portrait of Your Calf"; the eleventh "Portrait of Marianne;" the twelfth "Medusa." The series is not yet complete. I have only finished paintings four, five, six, and seven. The word *seer* occurred to me. In the sense Rimbaud used it. I love Lautréamont, Rimbaud, and Mácha over all others. They were all *seers*. Being a seer implies a *state of mind* whereby the poet, painter, etc. no longer desires to be revealed as a poet or painter. In short, he does not write, he does not paint. The poet seer cares little about creating art. And even less so an immortal Art. The poet seer is more interested in pursuing delight, a delight that endures during psychic creation. He is too indolent to put a poem down on paper. He considers it incidental. By way of explanation, we have Lautréamont's dictum : "Poetry must be made by all." The seer skirts along the border of death. When I wrote my biography of Rimbaud, I did not fully understand this word. It also has a different sense in the French.[37]

- **1940**

I have gotten over the biases of people and their opinions. Scholars cite Rimbaud as if his words should be taken literally. Break of day. That peculiar gloom before the change into morning. For the first time in many years I felt a yearning to walk through greenery, to hear the drone of forests and rivers. The magnificent song of birds in a beech wood. My nature is the nightclub with flora hardly rose-colored. I sit between Irena and Věra. And yet even I loved youth, flowers, spring, pink clouds in a pale blue sky, but this was long ago. Your miraculous summer body! Break of day. I have only Irena and Věra for company. I have never transgressed with them, and this is why they're fond of me. I enclose them in a web, like an old spider spinning its idea of life. There were other girls. They were clerks, dancers, philosophers, models, married women, and many others. These occasional lovers were not malign, they helped me bear my human squalor. A woman I knew before we met reminds me of you. I wanted to pay Marianne. Of course it was pointless. She didn't know how to clasp her hands in

37 Jindřich Štyrský, *Život J.A. Rimbauda. Dopisy a dokumenty* [The Life of J.A. Rimbaud: Letters and Documents], Edice Odeon, no. 62 (Prague: Jan Fromek, 1930). This was the first monograph in Czech on Rimbaud and his work.

devotion behind my neck and grunt on my shoulder when climaxing like you. She didn't have your ability to take wing like Nike of Samothrace straight to the moon. A person of greatness always seeks out and finds in life another who is great. Yesenin had Duncan, Maeterlinck had Leblanc, Degas had Sarah Bernhardt, Delacroix had Rachel, Bakst had Gzovska, whereas I had a cow confessing all in the pages of *Prague Girl*.[38] Evidently I am not a great man. I will never forget the time you told me after a torrid session in my bed that I only ever write you claptrap. Did you want me to write : I shall provide you with a monthly allowance of 3,000 crowns? Clearly you felt it too little when I wrote instead : . . . let the waves of love wash over me, and I think : Don't sink under the weight of your feelings, be glad you have a woman by your side in your tempestuous century, be proud you're able to love her. The fact that this woman even exists should be a pillar for you. You have to be worthy of her . . . If you win her affections, and she will love you, your life will be hers and your work will always be part of her. You will then finally have your Muse! . . . This Muse thoroughly wore me down. What should I do? I cross my legs. Love brings only indignity to the heart and memories. Broken youth floats in houses, houses float in bedrooms, bedrooms float in linen closets. All of it bathed in light. Memory and recollections each in turn play the role of executioner. And yet as separate entities they are instruments of the guilty, instruments of the innocent, standing idle. Solitude. The only reliable affection is that of friendship. Only barbarians rape the doves in Stromovka Park. A polychromatic portrait with a tiepin on a poster. Scapin in Hamlet's lavatory, my father in the role of Bacchus and my sister as Barborka. An opportunity to shampoo my hair like Lorelei. To perform, dance, play, identify with the nomad, with camels. [. . .]

Today I see her playing the diva, chasing popularity, publicity. Her perverse mind has gained the upper hand over good. She soon became a fixture in the Czech theater world that I find so repulsive. Where is her character? Perhaps you have worked your way up so high you'll become a housemaid of the spirit. The hunger for tawdry success

38 *Pražanka, List paní a dívek* [Prague Girl, a Journal for Women and Girls] was published by Rodina from 1924 to 1943, when the publishing house ceased to exist and its publisher, Artur Vaňous, was arrested by the Gestapo and sent to a concentration camp.

desires publicity, not immortality, popularity, not glory. Wretched Praline, you shall find success just like all those Ferbasovás and Baarovás,[39] and I wanted you to be my Sarah Bernhardt. Grand style! But you were born for the middle class. Imprudent Marianne. You'll never understand this : You will accuse me of envy and so forth all because you've forgotten to cast a critical eye on matters, on your profession, your art. You indulge in the fantasy of your brilliance, all the while you're sinking low. I recognized this when you told me of your wish to have your photo on the front page of *Illustrated Weekly,*[40] but that it cost 500 crowns. You implied that I should give it a go, that you would repay me. Your patron! It made me ill. Where might such pathological career ambition lead? It was clear to me this was an offer you'd extend to anyone. A demon keeps whispering in your ear : Now is your time! Now success is yours for the taking! You forget the year is 1940. You're getting lost in the crowd. I now think the only reason you were in a relationship with me was that you supposed I would help your career. When you recognized your mistake, your love cooled. You latched onto Mr. Mikota,[41] who arranged for you many front pages in the Czech press. I feel sorry for him, a great deal, but I wish you well with him! All in all I couldn't give a fig about who now commands your affections.

- **1940**

I have never run from the excesses of love, so I have never found peace in uncertainty. Many years ago I kept vigil over a dying man, over his labored breathing. I wished for death to end his agony, to sever my gaze that was incapable on its own of moving off him. Thousands of images rotate through the human eye daily. Yet my eyes was bereft of any expression of compassion. The man was my father. I also kept vigil over my mother. She had become so gaunt, skin and bones, before she died her wedding ring

39 Věra Ferbasová (1913–76), Czech film actress; Lída Baarová (1914–2000), Czech actress and mistress of Nazi propaganda minister Joseph Goebbels.

40 *Pestrý týden* was published from November 2, 1926, until April 28, 1945, that is, it ended with the war. Though noted for the high quality of its writing and photojournalism (akin to *Life* magazine), Štyrský is disparaging it as purely a commercial publication.

41 Václav Mikota (1896–1982), editor of *Hudba a národ* [Music and the Nation] (1940).

slipped off her finger. It rolled across the floor and fell over under the wardrobe. I have never been so painfully aware of my loneliness as then. Since that time I have grown close to many people. I don't know if they became alienated from me or if it was I who became alienated from them. Presumably I expect too much from life. I have experienced death once already and do not fear it. Death is nothing more than falling asleep. Ultimately I have the right to be ruthless, and I consider it a duty to nail to the pillory the names of the deserters, the names of all those who turned traitor. And not for the present, because I have no illusions about the Czech character of today, but for posterity. I see degeneration everywhere I look. In itself this is hardly remarkable, what is remarkable has been the SPEED of this degeneration. In poetry : at the moment patriotism is fashionable. Poets line their pockets with patriotism. Only when this love of homeland wears off, which I estimate will take an entire generation, will poetry again move toward the universal, will it be assessed by universal criteria : French and German : Goethe and Baudelaire. One who is no longer young loves youth. I have read nearly every collection put out by younger poets but have found nothing in them other than convention, verbal musicality, and saccharine verse. These young poets take themselves for militants, yet no one has informed them that they are fighting for something our generation long ago conquered and abandoned. For that matter, today's literary critics seem to me like crazy surveyors who have placed "our Czech spinning wheel" on their geodetic instruments. I know a single young poet, Jindřich Heisler, I know his poems and texts (published by Albert Skira in Paris to accompany Toyen's series of drawings *Les Spectres du désert*), who is the only one at present to have resisted the scent of printer's ink.

And my generation? They will be penning their *slave* songs until their dying days. František Halas, in your . . . poetic biography . . . of Božena Němcová you failed to mention when she got her first period! And Seifert has likewise commercialized his love of country in the most moronic way imaginable. Next to them Konstantin Biebl is no more than an afterthought, so why even bother with him. And Nezval? *Business is business!*[42] Where to find refuge? In the paradise of my childhood. This fetid Prague

[42] In English in the original.

has already devoured me. Where would I find refuge? In the realm of my childhood Arcadia or in dreams? A black snow falls from the clouds. My feet have drowned in the pavement. Hair has fallen in a mane from the cliffs. Eve dances in the middle of the street, her face lit by a cigarette. The Vltava weeps. The first drops of alcohol accumulate in vegetal wombs. And bile in livers. Eve received her first sweater from Adam. Eve had pale blue eyes, but she was *blind*. A bird described a circle, a bird with the long hair of Lorelei. Vibrating flowers and memories mixed with lentils and smoky smiles.[43] High moss. Small monkeys hidden behind broad leaves. Adam sat down next to Eve and masturbated. Thoughts are always mute. When God looked on this with his omnipresent eye he was shocked by Adam's behavior and put him to sleep. It's certainly no coincidence that Adam lost a rib while sleeping, and from that moment Eve had sight. Rosy plains. Brothel and harem signage. Gloves.

I, too, was once happy, and I launched myself from the springboard into the clouds. Yet I always leapt into the mirror. I did not drown in them. The knoll slightly opened. I saw maniacs. They darted through the streets, their hands filled with paintbrushes. A ball of white meat rolled behind them like a white carriage. It would be foolish to ask today what is happening in the guts of this moron. I suppose he contentedly digests whatever his belly has concocted. Only the brevity of life prevents me from opening again the books of this pedant of his obscene belly, this doubled-chinned beneficiary of Czech culture, whose sallow face with the purplish veins of an old lush resembles a dirty gourd. Once my friends resembled *casks*. A cask is an awesome thing. I love casks. Wine flows from them. Now these folks resemble *tubs,* dripping beer, and only plum slops flow from them. Imagine these large and small tubs : V. Nezval, J. Seifert, F. Halas, K. Biebl, E.F. Burian, B. Brouk, et al.[44] Beer nation! It's depressing. In such

43 An allusion to the "Cinderella" folk tale.

44 František Halas (1901–49), a poet active in avant-garde publications and a member of Devětsil; Konstantin Biebl (1898–1951), an avant-garde poet and member of Devětsil and the Surrealist Group; Emil František Burian (1904–59), an actor, playwright, and director influenced by Dada, Futurism, and Poetism, was a key member of Devětsil and collaborated with the group's Liberated Theater before founding his own leftist-oriented D34 theater in 1933; Bohuslav Brouk (1912–78) was a founding member of the Surrealist Group of Czechoslovakia who wrote extensively on psychoanalysis and sexual behavior.

dreary times it would be far better to be one of the wretched rabble than a member of this nation. The glutton is celebrating his fortieth birthday. For the occasion he has reworked Abbé Prévost's *Manon Lescaut,* divesting it of the original's genius. And E.F. Burian, another imbecile, scoundrel, and professional fraud is staging it as "Nezval's Manon." I cannot imagine anything more moronic. And the mob, that is, the Czech nation, squeals with delight, brays and grunts. MANON rhymes with MAMMON. Prévost doubly overcooked. Intercourse between genius and two celebrated sauciers. One cretin's versifying under the other's pathetic direction. Ripping off Meyerhold : *The Lady of the Camellias.*[45] Two chameleons have come together. I'm not going to comment further on such an awful production. I took off at the second intermission.

• **1940**

Overcoming the most hideous revulsion, I have started to write again. During the time I was in daily contact with Nezval my attitude toward him fluctuated between curiosity and contempt. Now I consider him a shit. You shit! You would've been better off reworking *The Ironmaster* by Georges Ohnet[46] than the tragic, tender Manon! I find it so fusty I'm practically suffocating. So the boy from Biskoupky is celebrating his fortieth birthday.[47] It is splashed all over the newspapers. I'm filled with loathing when I remember this face. I know no one as morally and physically corrupt as him. It would take a hardened man to describe this odious glob of filth. I saw you at a performance of *Manon*. I noticed you hovering near me, how you wanted to extend your hand. I turned away from you in disgust. I've been told you show up at every performance to collect your share of the take. You skinflint! Liar, I don't believe your patriotic fervor, your love for your native lump of dirt, because I know you like no one else knows you.

45 Vsevolod Emilevich Meyerhold (1874–1940), Russian theatre director, producer, and actor whose provocative experiments with physical being in unconventional settings were seminal for modern international theatre, staged *The Lady of the Camellias* (from the novel by Alexandre Duma, *fils*) in 1934.

46 *Le Maître des Forges* by Georges Ohnet (1848–1918), a novel and play both, has been persistently popular and few works of fiction have sold better in France. Ohnet wrote the story initially as a play, but no theater manager would stage it until it had first achieved success as a novel.

47 Vítězslav Nezval was born in 1900 in Biskoupky, Moravia.

You've never shown fervor for anything. You only feign enthusiasm in front of those folks who might be of some use to you. You even faked contempt. I remember the many times you sold me out for a glass of wine. And Teige, Toyen, Honzl, and all your closest friends? You were a poet, a great poet, therefore we forgave you everything. Now you're a shit! "O years of youth!" (Seifert). "Miss Gada-Nigi!"[48] Beyond the forest of windows. Beyond the forest.

I've idled away many moments at the feet of women, women with nails
carmine and orange
        but their touch never made me quiver
        never filled me with such delight
                                        as to kiss the arch
                                        of your foot
        women and stars
                buried by the rain   of this summer

I smile not tears   pearls strung on a necklace of laughter
        I know I am mute before you!

                                        Solitude is a terrible adventure!

Quite sad, my gray beauty, slender phantom,
noble bird of paradise, doleful movements languorously.

48 "Miss Gada-Nigi" is a poem by Jaroslav Seifert that first appeared in *Disk* (Prague: 1923), 6. Nezval's "Abeceda" and Štyrský's concrete poem "Obraz" appeared in the same issue.

TRANSLATOR'S NOTE

The three sections comprising *Dreamverse* represent the majority of Jindřich Štyrský's writing. The original Czech editions of "Dreams" (*Sny*, 1970, republished by Argo in 2003) and "Verse" (*Poesie*, 1946), both published posthumously, have been translated in their entirety ("Alcohol and a Rose" was published earlier, in 1924, and does not appear in the 1946 collection). The "Writings" section draws on the volume of collected texts edited by Lenka Bydžovská and Karel Srp, simply titled *Texty* (Argo, 2007), which expands on their 1996 edition where some of these texts appeared for the very first time. We have not, however, included everything, leaving out numerous book, magazine, theater, and exhibition reviews, short articles on Fantômas, František Bidlo's drawings, and Bohuslav Brouk, a brief overview on Rimbaud's life and work, longer biographical essays on Marquis de Sade, and arguably Štyrský's most famous text, "Emilie Comes to Me in a Dream," which Twisted Spoon Press has published in *Edition 69*. Despite the many repetitions, or because of them, as they indicate what Štyrský considered important enough to reuse or rework, all the Artificialist texts have been translated. The Introduction by Karel Teige was originally written for a monograph on Štyrský that was prohibited from publication after the Communist Party's February 1948 coup in Czechoslovakia.

The numbered footnotes for "Writings" are my own, and they are selective, not comprehensive. For the most part, they are provided to explain some of the more obscure persons, places, publications, events, or historical references, especially when they pertain to interwar Czechoslovakia. The asterisked notes in "Dreams" are the author's, and in most cases were added later parenthetically than when the dream occurred or was recorded. Many are dated to 1941, which would suggest they are some of the very last additions to the book's final form.

Štyrský had *Dreams* largely complete by the end of 1940 with a plan for its layout indicating which images were to be included and where. He then added the collage *The Pope of Czech Literature* in 1941 as a sardonic accompaniment to the text "Dream of Vítězslav Nezval." Since publication of the book was impossible under Nazi occupation, Štyrský printed up 150 pamphlet-sized copies of extracts as a kind of New Year's card for 1941 : included were six reproductions, the text "Dream of the Tiny Alabaster Hand," and longer citations on dreams from Lichtenberg and Nerval. When Štyrský died suddenly in 1942 (he had a chronic heart condition), the manuscript and layout plan for *Dreams* as well as the rest of his unpublished writings and other assorted work were saved by Toyen. This enabled the first publication in 1970 of the book in its entirety following Štyrský's original conception.

Given the personal, hermetic nature of his work, it seems Štyrský had intended to write an afterword introduced by the image "The Key to Dreams," appearing here at the very beginning, but since he never got around to it before his death, the editor of the first publication, the renowned art historian František Šmejkal, wrote one instead, noting : "Although for some of the more hermetic dreams we are lacking explanations, a key such as knowledge of some of Štyrský's experiences from waking life would provide, this does not mean the entire book is an indecipherable enigma for us. Just the opposite. Many facts from his life that had a decisive influence on the form and latent content of his dreams are known to us from his contemporaries, while other clues can be found in his poetry and theoretical texts, and ultimately many of the dreams are rendered in enough vividness on the pages of this book so as to require no further information." Indeed, the cross-referencing between the three sections of this volume and the repurposing of bits of text should help the reader at least to some extent penetrate Štyrský's thinking. One such example is the trauma he experienced at age six when his half-sister Marie died (she was twenty-one), and she subsequently recurs in myriad guises : as the first image of "Dreams" and then throughout all his writing in transmuted form as Emilie, Klára, and other "women-phantoms."

The three-part "A Generation's Corner" might be Štyrský's most consequential essay. Written over 1929-30, it sparked a vigorous debate among the Czech avant-garde, and some of the reaction can be gleaned by Štyrský's responses in parts II and III and in the short statement "I am not, nor have I ever been . . ." ("Brief Prolegomena" should also be read as part of this context). I decided to present "A Generation's Corner" as a single text for clarity, though each part appeared in a different issue of *Odeon* (cf. the bibliography). While the full context is absent, the ensuing brouhaha pulled in not only Karel Teige and Julius Fučík, but Vladislav Vančura, Vítězslav Nezval, Záviš Kalandra, and a host of other artists and communist hacks, launching a decades-long debate on the relationship of art and the avant-garde to Communism in general and to the Soviet Union more specifically, especially as the 1930s wore on and the totalitarian nature of Stalinism became harder to ignore. Yet even by late 1929, when Štyrský penned his text, many things were already coming to a head for progressive Czech artists : Vančura and six other prominent writers — among them Josef Hora, Ivan Olbracht, and Jaroslav Seifert — quit the Communist Party of Czechoslovakia in protest to its hard-line Bolshevization and subservience to Comintern directives; Teige publicly berated Vančura for quitting the Party and then accepting the State Prize for Literature (for *The Last Judgment*); ever more aggressive censorship by Czechoslovak authorities led to the confiscation of the first Czech translation of Lautréamont's *Les Chants de Maldoror,* for which Štyrský had created "illustrations"; the Left Front was established as an organization of the Czechoslovak "progressive intelligentsia" with Štyrský as a founding member. And then at the end of the following year the Second Conference of Revolutionary Writers took place in Kharkov, Ukraine, and leftist artists were expected to toe the Party line on the creation and promotion of "proletarian art and literature." But this and the subsequent attacks on the avant-garde as bourgeois at its core left many artists none too sanguine about where their continued affiliation with communist organizations might lead them. The rifts that developed in these years continued through the founding of the Surrealist Group of Czechoslovakia in 1934 and the serious schism that developed between, mainly, Nezval and everyone else in 1938. Some of this informs the venom Štyrský directs at Nezval in the text fragments dated to 1940.

Štyrský concisely summed up his views on the art-politics-society nexus in a talk given for a seminar held by Jan Mukařovský in Prague in winter 1938, presumably around the time the Surrealist Group of Czechoslovakia was about to splinter : "And yet I admit that poetry and painting are adventure enough for my life and I have no desire whatsoever to participate in the daily political madhouse. My art conveys no idea that would interest the general public of today. I cannot say that this pleases me, because I do not like feeling isolated, but isolation is definitely more preferable if it is away from the convention of the masses, from the political haggling, from the corruption in art, from the general treachery, and from having to traffic with this nation, more preferable even than the popularity one might attain by doing all these things, and therefore it is something I hold in contempt."

Finally, a brief word on the vignettes that accompany each section title : **SNY** is Štyrský's original titling from the first edition; the bat with a bouquet of lilies of the valley for "Verse" was the cover image for the first edition of *Poesie* in 1946 — Štyrský said he was looking at lilies of the valley when he was told of his sister's death, so the flower became emblematic for him, a fetish even, and regularly pops up in his work; the image for "Writings" is *Madame Mazepa* (1939, pen and ink and collage).

I have tried to retain as much of Štyrský's stylistic quirks in both his poetry and prose as feasible, though, as with any translation, concessions had to be made for the sake of intelligibility. My heartfelt gratitude goes to Misha Sidenberg for helping to untangle some of the more knotty and convoluted passages, to Bruno Solařík for vetting the translation, pointing out misreadings, and otherwise making numerous excellent suggestions, and to the Ministry of Culture of the Czech Republic for seeing their way to support this project. Any poetic license taken too liberally or mistranslations that remain are of course my own doing.

Jed Slast
Prague, 2018

BIBLIOGRAPHY

"Introduction" by Karel Teige originally published as "Jindřich Štyrský." In *Poesie*, Jindřich Štyrský, edited by Alena Nádvorníková, 47-53. Prague: Československý spisovatel, 1992.

DREAMS

Sny (1925–1940), edited and afterword by František Šmejkal. Prague: Odeon, 1970.

VERSE

First published in *Poesie*. Knižnice Kvartu, edited by Vít Orbtel, vol.1. Prague: B. Stýblo, 1946; republished by Československý spisovatel in 1992. The collection does not include "Alcohol and a Rose," which was published as "Alkohol a růže." *Pásmo* 1, no. 1 (March 1924): 6.

WRITINGS

All texts in this section have been selected from their latest republication in Jindřich Štyrský. *Texty,* edited by Lenka Bydžovská and Karel Srp. Prague: Argo, 2007. The original publication dates and sources are given below.

"From a Lecture at Masaryk University in Brno" : "Z přednášky na Masarykově univerzitě v Brně dne 9.4.1925." In *Štyrský a Toyen 1921–1945*, 20-21. Brno: Moravská galerie, 1966.

"A Popular Introduction to Artificialism" : "Populární uvedení do artificielismu." In *Fronta. Mezinárodní sborník soudobé aktivity*, 18. Brno: Edition Fronta, 1927.

"Artificialism" : "Artificielisme." *ReD* 1 (October 1927): 28-30.

"Three Chapters from a Book in Progress" : "Tří kapitoly z připravované knihy." *Horizont* 1, no. 8 (October 1927): 134-135.

"The Poet" : "Básník. (Přednáška proslovená při vernisáži výstavy)." *Rozpravy Aventina* 3, no. 20 (June 6, 1928): 241-242.

"On Artificialism" : Undated manuscript, originally published as "Přednáška o artificielismu." In *Každý z nás stopuje svoji ropuchu. (Texty 1923–40)*, edited by Lenka Bydžovská and Karel Srp, 27-35. Prague: Thyrsus, 1996.

"A Generation's Corner" :
"Koutek generace [I]." *Odeon – Literární kurýr* 1, no. 1 (October 1929): 12.
"Koutek generace [II]." *Odeon – Literární kurýr* 1, no. 3 (December 1929): 45.
"Koutek generace [III]." *Odeon – Literární kurýr* 1, no. 4 (January 1930): 60.

"I am not, nor have I ever been . . ." : "Nebyl jsem a nejsem . . ." *Tvorba* 4/2, no. 24 (1929): 380.

"The Drawings of Writers" : "Kresby literátů." *Odeon – Literární kurýr* 1, no. 5 (Feb. 1930): 68-69.

"On the Štyrský & Toyen Exhibition" : "Poznámka k výstavě Štyrského a Toyen." *Musaion*, no. 11 (April 1930): 241-243.

"Recent Books" : "Knihy." *Odeon – Literární kurýr* 1, no. 7 (April 1930): 103-104 and no. 8 (May 1930): 126.

"On Painting" : "K obrazům." *Kvart* 1, no. 1 (spring 1930): 36-37.

"Brief Prolegomena" : "Malá prolegomena." *Rok – Kulturní leták* (October 1931): 1, 4.

"An Inspired Illustrator" : "Inspirovaná ilustrátorka." In *Almanach Kmene, 1932–33*, edited by František Halas, 71-74. Prague: Kmen, 1932.

"The Joys of a Book Illustrator" : "Radosti ilustrátora knih." In *Jarní Almanach Kmene – Jízdní řád literatury a poesie*, edited by Adolf Hoffmeister, 128-130. Prague: Kmen, 1932.

"The Painter Who Draws: Man with a Flaming Mane!" : "Kreslící malíř, toť muž s hořící hřívou!" *Listy pro umění a kritiku* 1, no. 1 (February 15, 1933): 26-27.

"Flashback : Toyen's Spring Postcards" : "Vzpomínka. K vydání jarních pohlednic DP od Toyen." *Panorama* 11, no. 2 (March 25, 1933): 28-29.

"The Landscape of Marquis de Sade" : "Kraj Markýze de Sade." *Rozpravy Aventina* 9, no. 1 (Sept. 27, 1933): 6.

"Surrealist Painting" : "Surrealistické malířství (Několik poznámek)." *Doba* 1, no. 9 (May 24, 1934): 135-136.

"Surrealist Photography" : "Surrealistická fotografie." *České slovo* 27, no. 10 (Jan. 30, 1935): 10.

"The Importance of Emil Filla" : "Fillův význam." In *Emil Filla*, 9-10. Brno: V. Jelínek and F. Venera, 1936.

"One who is no longer young . . ." : "Člověk, který už není mlád . . ." In Vladimír Holan. *Bagately*. Sebrané spisy Vladimíra Holana, edited by Vladimír Justl, vol. X, 370-371. Prague: Odeon, 1988. Response to a survey on the modern poet and poetry conducted by V. Holan and dated December 20, 1939.

"Assorted Text Fragments" : "Fragmenty z pozůstalosti." *Revolver Revue*, no. 26 (September 1994): 335-339; reprinted in *Každý z nás stopuje svoji ropuchu. (Texty 1923–40)*, 187-195. Prague: Thyrsus, 1996.

JINDŘICH ŠTYRSKÝ (Dolní Čermná, 1899–Prague, 1942) was a painter, poet, editor, photographer, and collagist. His outstanding and varied oeuvre also included numerous book covers and illustrations. He also wrote studies of both Rimbaud and Marquis de Sade. He became a member of Devětsil in 1923, participating in their group exhibitions. Between 1928–29 he was director of the group's drama wing, the "Liberated Theater," where he collaborated with Vítězslav Nezval among others. Štyrský was also an active editor. In addition to his Edition 69 series, he edited the *Erotic Review,* which he launched in 1930, and *Odeon,* where many of his shorter texts appeared. He was a founding member of the Surrealist Group of Czechoslovakia.

KAREL TEIGE (1900–51) was a Czech avant-garde artist, cover designer, writer, critic, and theoretician. He was a founding member of both Devětsil in 1920 and the Surrealist Group of Czechoslovakia in 1934. Author of the Manifesto of Poetism and many theoretical essays, Teige's major works include *The Minimum Dwelling, The Laughing World* (and its companion volume *The Fragrant World*), and *Surrealism against the Current*. Fearing arrest after being labeled an "enemy of the people" by the Communist Party of Czechoslovakia, he died of a heart attack in 1951.

JED SLAST is a native of Richmond, Virginia, and has resided in Prague since 1991. His translations include *Edition 69*, *A Prague Flâneur*, and *The Transformations of Mr. Hadlíz*.

DREAMVERSE
by Jindřich Štyrský

Translated from the original Czech
by Jed Slast

Introduction by Karel Teige
Design by Silk Mountain
Typeset in Garamond Pro

FIRST EDITION 2018

TWISTED SPOON PRESS
P.O. Box 21
150 21 Prague 5
Czech Republic
www.twistedspoon.com
info@twistedspoon.com

IMAGE TO WORD 3

Printed and bound in the Czech Republic by PB Tisk

Distributed to the trade by

CENTRAL BOOKS
www.centralbooks.com

SCB DISTRIBUTORS
www.scbdistributors.com

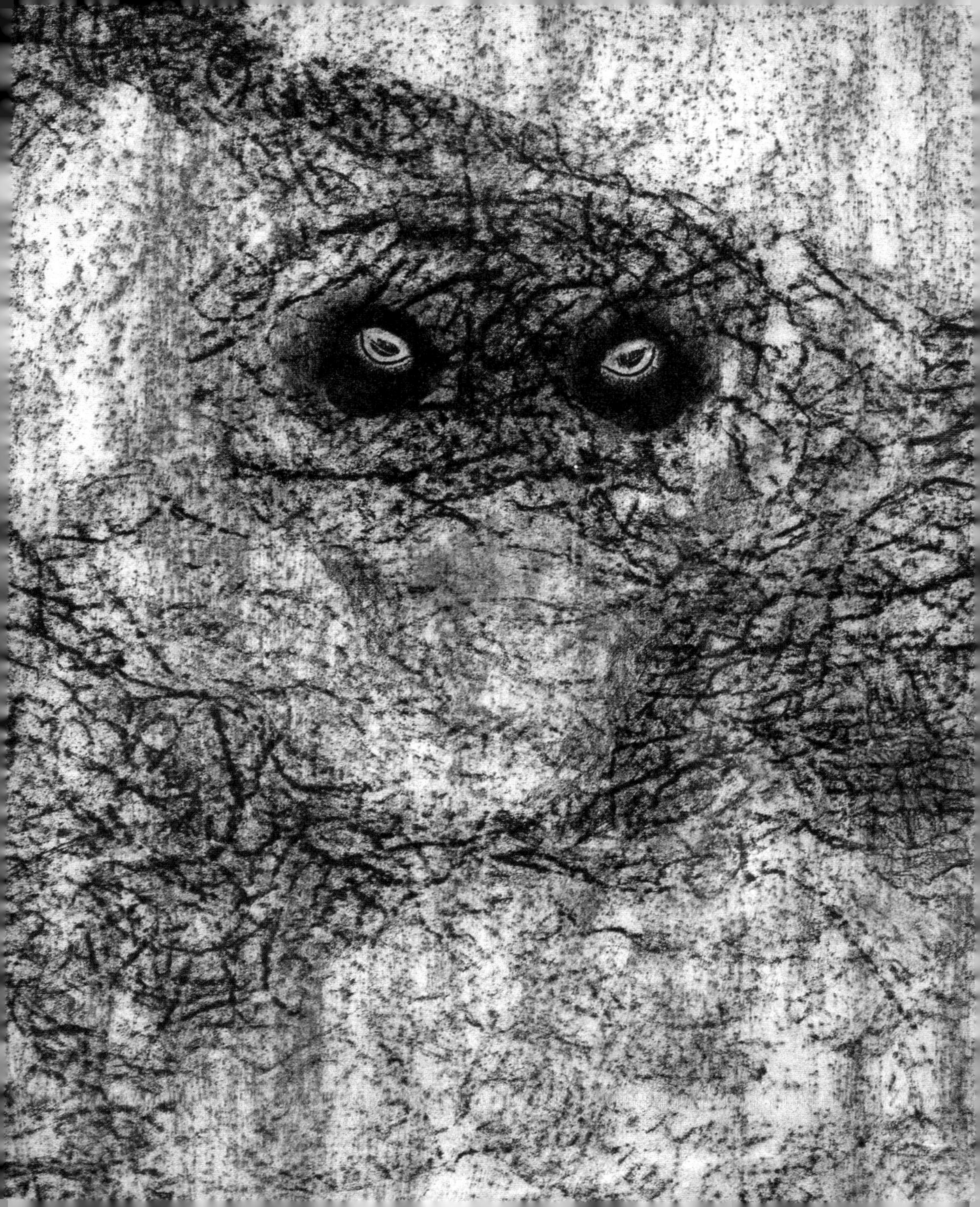